Dr. John A. MacDonald, M.D., was a practicing surgeon, teacher, and cancer specialist before undergoing his own operations for heart disease and cancer. This book, completed shortly before his death, stands as a fitting memorial to a man whose life was devoted to the care and cure of others.

John A. MacDonald, M.D.
Facing the scalpel

WHAT TO EXPECT, WHAT TO BEWARE OF WHEN YOU HAVE AN OPERATION

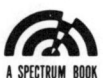

PRENTICE-HALL, INC., *Englewood Cliffs, N. J. 07632*

Library of Congress Cataloging in Publication Data

MACDONALD, JOHN A (date)
   Facing the scalpel.

   (A Spectrum Book)
   Includes bibliographical references and index.
   1. Surgery—Popular works. I. Title.
RD31.3.M33   1981   617   81-341
ISBN 0-13-299198-5   AACR1
ISBN 0-13-299180-2 (pbk.)

Editorial/production supervision and
interior design by Carol Smith
Cover design by Michael Aron
Manufacturing buyer: Cathie Lenard

Originally published under the title *Undergoing Surgery*
by McClelland and Stewart Limited,
25 Hollinger Road, Toronto M4B 3G2, Canada.
Copyright © 1980 by Madeleine MacDonald.

U.S.A. Edition, *Facing the Scalpel,*
© 1981 by Prentice-Hall, Inc., *Englewood Cliffs, New Jersey 07632*

A SPECTRUM BOOK

All rights reserved. No part of this book may be
reproduced in any form or by any means
without permission in writing from the publisher.

10 9 8 7 6 5 4 3 2 1

Printed in the United States of America

PRENTICE-HALL INTERNATIONAL INC., *London*
PRENTICE-HALL OF AUSTRALIA, PTY. LIMITED, *Sydney*
PRENTICE-HALL OF CANADA, LTD., *Toronto*
PRENTICE-HALL OF INDIA PRIVATE LIMITED, *New Delhi*
PRENTICE-HALL OF JAPAN, INC., *Tokyo*
PRENTICE-HALL OF SOUTHEAST ASIA PTE. LTD., *Singapore*
WHITEHALL BOOKS LIMITED, *Wellington, New Zealand*

Contents

PREFACE, *vii*

INTRODUCTION, *1*

1 THE ANNOUNCEMENT:
YOU NEED AN OPERATION, *8*

2 THE DIAGNOSIS, *17*

3 HOW TO PICK YOUR SURGEON, *34*

4 CHOOSING YOUR HOSPITAL, *48*

5 MEETING YOUR SURGEON:
THE VERBAL CONTRACT, *59*

6 ENTERING THE HOSPITAL:
THE PREOPERATIVE PERIOD, *75*

7 THE OPERATION, *89*

8 THE POSTOPERATIVE EXPERIENCE, *103*

9 FROM PATIENT TO LITIGANT, *115*

10 HOW TO REDUCE MALPRACTICE SUITS, *137*

INDEX, *145*

Preface

I used to think, as my surgical experience grew and I became increasingly aware of the complexities of the medical world, that I had developed an objective yet compassionate overview of the doctor-patient relationship. As a general surgeon I have performed a great variety of surgical procedures, from removing toenails and hemorrhoids to bowel and liver resections. I have taught medical students, interns, and surgical residents for nearly 20 years, and have served as an expert witness in close to 500 medico-legal examinations, acting for the plaintiff and the defendant in nearly equal numbers.

However, I have recently gained more insight by being a patient than in all my years of medical school and practice. During the past three years I have experienced both open-heart surgery and the removal of part of one lung for cancer. These operations have given me a new perspective; I now know what it is like to be at the other end of the scalpel.

We doctors seem to forget that, for many patients, an operation is the most important event of their lives. We forget that they must endure this awesome experience, immersed in the mysteries of life and death helplessly anesthetized and utterly alone.

I have come to appreciate that a patient's reasons for agreeing to surgery may be vastly different from those of his doctor, and that there is both truth and urgency in the adage that "operations are for the patient, not for the surgeon." Were we to apply these criteria to our patients, there would be far fewer unnecessary operations. Dr. John Hunter, the eminent eighteenth-century surgeon, was deeply aware of the blindness of many doctors to the patient's point of view, when he counselled the surgeons of his day, "Never perform an operation on another that you would not have performed on yourself."

As doctors and patients we should heed Doctor Hunter.

Introduction

More and more people in the United States will have a surgical operation this year. Many of these operations will be planned, but a large number will not. With the rising population, especially of the aged, there will be more surgical procedures in this high-risk group. Both heart disease and cancer are on the rise: Approximately 400,000 open-heart operations for coronary artery disease will be done this year in the United States alone. Cancer is increasing at a rate of over 1 percent per year, and the preferred method of primary treatment of the five most common cancers—lung, colon and rectum, breast, pancreas, and stomach—is surgery.* Most of these operations will be elective surgery, in the nonemergency category.

Emergency surgical procedures—often secondary to trauma—will also increase in number. Automobile accidents are the principal source of trauma in North America, but gunshot and stab wounds are not far behind as the incidence of violence continues to rise in most cities in the

---

*Skin cancer is the most common variety, but it does not rank with these five as a major cause of death from the disease.

2 Introduction

region. Surgeons in many hospitals are kept busy specializing in trauma alone.

Also, in our image-oriented society, there has been a proliferation of rejuvenating procedures to ameliorate the effects of aging. To enhance our presentability, we are resorting to cosmetic procedures at an ever-increasing rate (particularly face-lifts, tummy tucks, breast augmentation by silicone implants, and nose bobs, or rhinoplasty, to improve the configuration of the nose). These cosmetic operations can keep a plastic surgeon fully occupied and his or her bank account straining at the seams.

A byproduct of our increasing population has been a corresponding rise in the number of doctors and surgeons and an alarming increase in the percentage of unnecessary operations.* The problem has been recognized and publicized by a U.S. House of Representatives subcommittee and is of grave concern to the American College of Surgeons. The percentage of unnecessary operations has been pegged as high as 26 percent. The fatalities resulting from the operations have resulted in the disturbing figure of 10,000 in the United States alone, with a cost of $4 billion.†

Hysterectomy and planned cesarean section have become two of the leading operations in the category termed "unnecessary." It is not surprising, then, that hysterectomy also heads the list of operations that result in the highest incidence of malpractice litigation. Abortion is now ap-

---

*According to *Time,* May 28, 1979, the number of physicians in the United States has grown from 1.5 per 1,000 in 1960 to 2 per 1,000 in 1978. The distribution of surgeons is also of concern—40 per 100,000 in urban areas and 20 per 100,000 in rural areas (*American College of Surgeons Bulletin,* March 1976). In total, there were 437,000 physicians in the United States in 1978, of whom 342,000 were involved in patient care.

†House Interstate and Foreign Commerce's Oversight and Investigations subcommittee, headed by Rep. John E. Moss (Calif.), revised report, 1977.

proved by the laws of the land. Increasingly, it has become a procedure used for contraception rather than a method to protect the physical and mental well-being of a pregnant woman. The legitimized abortion clinic is now an established entity.

As a result of all this surgical activity, the staggering hospital costs and surgical fees will be in the billions in the United States. In the province of Ontario, Canada, with a universal health scheme, the costs are on the rampage and cannot be met solely by the paid premiums of the insured. The deficits must be met from the general treasury. An announced premium increase to meet these deficits was defeated in the legislature.

An unpleasant consequence of the increasing number of operations in all areas has been a rising volume of malpractice suits. The courts in the United States are swamped with a backlog of cases. Awards to injured parties are astronomical. Lawyers' fees, some arrived at on a contingency basis, (i.e., in proportion to the awards) have contributed to the mounting costs. Malpractice insurance premiums in the United States are nearly prohibitive, as high as $50,000 per year for high-risk specialties such as anesthesia and orthopedics. Some insurance carriers have abandoned the field of medical malpractice altogether. And many surgeons in desperation have refused to take out any malpractice insurance at all, adopting the attitude, "Let the patient take the risk." If successfully sued, they declare bankruptcy or maintain that everything is in their spouses' names.

In a society that is compensation conscious, that demands redress for any and every loss or injury, the surgical complication is an obvious target for justice under our adversary system. A patient has an operation, develops a complication, suffers pain and loss of income, and therefore demands recompense for pain, suffering, and economic loss. The concept of no-fault insurance, whereby such claims could be handled without resort to the courts, appeals to many people, though lawyers are not among them for obvious reasons (see Chapter 10).

This book was undertaken to enlighten a prospective patient on what to expect when he or she has an operation; to define the inherent risks of surgery; and to answer some commonly asked questions: What is an act of malpractice or negligence, and what is simply bad luck? When might one expect to be recompensed for personal injury? How can one find out beforehand, short of going to a lawyer and paying heavy legal fees, that one has an insupportable claim?

It was written also as a guide on how to choose a surgeon, hospital, or clinic (when you have a choice); how to avoid an unnecessary operation; and, most importantly, how to avoid a disaster.

Today, people give more consideration to their choice of tailor or hairdresser than they do to the selection of their surgeon. Is it any wonder, then, that malpractice claims are on the rise, when expectations are greater than the actual results, or when there has been an unanticipated complication?

I hope that this book will help to pinpoint some of the causes of rising litigation and at the same time will suggest means to reduce unnecessary, fruitless lawsuits.

As a general surgeon, I have performed a broad spectrum of surgical procedures—from toenails and hemorrhoids to bowel and liver resections; I have also taught medical students, interns, and surgical residents for nearly twenty years. But I have gained more insight on these problems as a patient over the past three years than during all my years of medical school and practice. For I have had two major operations—open-heart surgery for coronary-artery disease, and a lobectomy (excision of part of one lung) for cancer.

These operations have given me a new perspective in

all aspects of the doctor–patient relationship—from receiving the diagnosis, through the decision-making process of the need for surgery, and on into the postoperative and recovery periods. I have a greater understanding now of what it is like to be a patient—at the other end of the scalpel. I have come to appreciate through this experience the attitudes and concerns expressed by patients who are about to undergo a major operation. For many, an operation is the most important event in their lives. The mysteries of life and death surround it. One is so utterly helpless under anesthesia—and the event must be faced entirely alone.

I have come to appreciate that the indications for surgery for doctors ourselves are often different than those for patients. There is truth to the adage that "operations are for patients, not for surgeons." Were we to apply the same criteria to our patients as to ourselves, there might well be fewer unnecessary operations performed. As Dr. John Hunter so aptly expressed it: "Never perform an operation on another that you would not have performed on yourself." What better criterion for the need for surgery?

As a general surgeon, I have had experience as an expert witness in close to 500 medicolegal examinations performed at the request of lawyers. I have acted both for the plaintiff and for the defense in nearly equal numbers. (I have always tried to preserve my objectivity and independence from what might be construed as "pressure.") Therefore, I have had a long interest in medicolegal problems. I am also concerned by the malpractice situation.

The malpractice situation in Canada has not yet reached the crisis proportions that exist in the United States. The trend, though, is moving in that direction. There is usually a ten-year lag in Canada for most sociological changes. The national atmosphere, sociologically and politically, has probably contributed to the malpractice morass in the United States. Consumer's groups are numerous and aggressive; Proposition 13, which would hardly get off the ground in Canada, passed in California. There was Watergate, with its interplay of investigative reporting, Grand Jury hearings, Senate subcommittees, judicial inquiry for impeachment of the President, resulting in his ultimate resignation. Americans are fascinated by litigation—for civil rights amendments against discrimination by virtue of race or sex; for libel, divorce, cohabitation, separation, and equal rights for gays!! They have Nader's Raiders, class actions by consumer groups all seeking redress in court against government or giant corporations. The media (press, radio and TV) give them extensive coverage. Lawyers can readily be found who will champion a cause for a contingency fee—in fact will advertise for clients who are disenchanted with the promised results of surgical operations. And in the United States everyone has a constitutional right to a trial by jury. And juries tend to be sympathetic to plaintiffs rather than to defendants (surgeons).

Then, too, the image people see of the sympathetic doctor on "Marcus Welby" or the brilliant surgeon on "The Doctors" is not always what they meet in their local hospitals. Rather, their surgeon tends to be distant, uncommunicative, and superior, almost contemptuous of his patients, treating them as if they were imbeciles. On one recent poll of Americans that listed the professionals or occupations they most respected, doctors did make the list of the top ten! In England, physicians are held in the same esteem(?) as other health professionals—nurses, physiotherapists, and technicians.

The position in Canada today is analogous to that in the United States ten years ago.* If the trend continues in Canada, we *will* have a crisis in ten years; if it continues

---

*Hon. W. Z. Estey, BA, LLB, LLM, "Medical Litigation in Canada," *Canadian Journal of Surgery,* March 1978, *21,* pp. 156–170.

at its present rate in the United States, they will have a disaster!

This book should not be looked upon in any sense as a general indictment of doctors or surgeons. Most of the people I knew who practiced the art of surgery were honorable and decent human beings of great dedication. It is not to these surgeons that my remarks are directed; rather to those who perform the bulk of unnecessary surgery, who perform ghost surgery or other less than honorable practices. It is hoped that good surgeons will not be offended, for they have little cause to be; on the other hand, it is of little or no concern to me if the small percentage of poor surgeons are offended.

Let us examine the intricacies of a surgical operation, from the moment you are told you need one to the point in time when you have fully recovered. We consider the indications, the need for confirmation of the diagnosis, the advisability of a second opinion or consultation, the surgical contract—the consent form—the entire process from admission to the hospital to removal of the sutures. Last, we consider the potential complications that may occur—those that form part of the bargain, and those that do not. Failing complete recovery, we review the circumstances that may help you to determine whether you have a genuine grievance or not, one that warrants redress. Suggestions are made as to how the overall situation may be improved.

Only one person benefits if your operation turns out to be a disaster. It is not the surgeon, and it certainly isn't the patient; it can only be the lawyer or the undertaker. Let us then consider together a few of the ways to avoid some of the unheralded pitfalls when you are in need of an operation.

1 The announcement: you need an operation

In many instances, you will be told that you need an operation by your family physician. On occasion, the need will be self-evident—you have an enlarging hernia, your ulcer is no longer responding to treatment, your periods are becoming more and more irregular, the bleeding heavier and heavier. Perhaps it will be your gynecologist or your personal surgeon (if you have one) who gives you the news.

In cases of emergency, such as following an auto accident, in which you are unconscious or have internal injuries, you may not be told at all. You will be transported by ambulance and directed by police at the scene to the nearest hospital. In such cases you will have no choice of hospital or of surgeon. It will simply be a matter of luck and circumstance as to how well you fare. You can be assured, though, that in most hospitals handling trauma, there will be an adequate if not superb surgical staff. The bodies that control hospital accreditation have partly seen to this. Though the patient exercises little choice in this situation, and though lawsuits do result because of personal injury, they are more likely to be directed against the party who caused the accident and the injury than against the surgeon.

Nevertheless, many hospitals now employ full-time emergency personnel, doctors trained in emergency care who supervise all admissions to the emergency department. In the past, this care was often provided by the least-trained members of the hospital staff—interns and residents, but this is not so any longer. The trend is definitely toward highly trained medical and surgical personnel who devote their entire time and energy to the management of emergencies.

The majority of lawsuits directed against surgeons are in the area of elective operations (i.e., the hysterectomy, radiologic diagnostic procedures, and orthopedic procedures). Only one trauma-related operation places high on the list—open reduction of hip fractures—and this most often occurs from falls in elderly patients, not from car accidents.

Let us consider, then, only those procedures in which you do have an opportunity to review the need or to make a choice. It is necessary to define at the outset the various categories of operations from the standpoint of their urgency.

TYPES OF SURGERY

EMERGENCY The extreme emergencies—an automobile accident, a gunshot or stab wound, a brain injury, perforation of an organ or a ruptured aneurysm—fall into this category. In these situations, there is implied consent when you are presented to the emergency unit of a hospital. A patient in such circumstances will most often be unable to sign the consent form. Frequently there are relatives nearby who will assume this responsibility, but not always.

10 The announcement

In any case, someone other than the patient must sign the consent form—hence, the term *implied consent.*

URGENT   The urgent category is a situation of slightly less gravity—a bowel obstruction, acute appendicitis, an ectopic pregnancy, fetal distress, or a strangulated hernia. In these moderate emergencies, a patient is usually conscious and capable of decision and of signing his or her consent. Although there seldom is much choice, since delay could result in tragedy, there is still an element of participation in the decision, though few would be so cavalier as to ignore their surgeon's advice in such situations.

SEMIURGENT   The next category is the semiurgent one, which is only slightly less grave than the foregoing situations. Here we are dealing with cancers—of any organ—an inflamed gallbladder, a partial obstruction of the digestive tract, an unruptured aneurysm, and so forth. A situation in this category could suddenly become an emergency as a result, for example, of the sudden rupture of the gallbladder or aneurysm or from the gut obstruction's becoming complete. It may be somewhat artificial to make two separate categories of the urgent and semiurgent groups, but there are subtle distinctions. Again, the patient has a choice—he or she still may refuse to have the cancer treated by surgery and may opt for radiation or no treatment at all. But most patients in the semiurgent category consent willingly to surgery.

ELECTIVE   In the fourth category are the elective operations, by far the most common of all surgery. Most operations for gallstones (cholecystectomy) and hysterectomies fall into this group, as well as those for hernias, varicose veins, even open-heart and lung operations. For the elective procedure, time is not of the essence, and urgency is not usually a factor except when complications arise. Then, if the hernia becomes strangulated or obstructed, it falls by definition into the urgent group.

In this area there has usually been a preoperative period during which a diagnosis has been made, the indications for surgery reviewed, and the choice of surgeon and hospital discussed. There has been time to establish informed consent, or what amounts to a contractual arrangement between patient and surgeon.

The relative frequency of these categories may be gauged by a review of the admissions to a surgical service for a one-year period in a busy general hospital in a metropolitan center. In 1977, for the general surgical service of St. Michael's Hospital in Toronto, Canada, there were 936 elective admissions, 768 emergency admissions, and 45 classified as urgent or semiurgent. Thus a little more than half (53.5 percent) are in the elective category. In other subspecialties, the rate of elective operations is much higher.

In a similar category is the cosmetic procedure. This is almost always an elective operation. It is not done for therapeutic purposes—that is, to remove gallstones before they cause complications or to fix a hernia before it becomes strangulated. Rather, the cosmetic operation is performed solely to improve one's appearance—a nose bob, a breast implant, a face-lift, and so forth. Few of these can be considered to have *prophylactic* (i.e., designed to prevent disease) value unless one were to include such a procedure as varicose vein ligation, which might have *both* cosmetic and therapeutic objectives—improving the appearance of one's legs and preventing a complication such as phlebitis. It is in this area, where there is both informed consent and expectations of dramatic improvement, that many malpractice claims occur. The procedures contracted for often cost the patient an amount far in excess of many of those in the other categories. For example, a cosmetic breast augmentation using a silicone prosthesis may cost two to four times

12 The announcement

more than a modified radical mastectomy for cancer of the breast.

Some operations are simply optional. A man opts to have a vasectomy, a woman a tubal ligation. They are both elective procedures as well, though some may wish to define them as semiurgent, depending on the circumstances of the patient—risking an unwanted pregnancy, for example. They can hardly be called cosmetic. For clarity, it is useful to classify surgical operations from the standpoint of their magnitude as well—major, semimajor, and minor.

MAGNITUDE

MAJOR AND SEMIMAJOR SURGERY Few will quarrel with the definition of a major operation as one that represents a serious threat to life, or one with a high mortality rate or high morbidity (complication) rate. This area includes open-heart operations, lung operations, resections for cancer of the bowel, liver, pancreas, or kidney, and many others.

Some operations should be considered major even though they do not constitute a threat to life. They are of long duration and require exceptional facility in their performance. In this area are operations on the retina of the eye, inner-ear procedures, reimplantation of a digit or limb, and reconstructive operations, to name a few.

The semimajor procedures are those that constitute much less threat to life or are of much shorter duration than the aforementioned. Most orthopedic procedures, gallbladder operations, hysterectomies, and mastectomies fall into this category. The mortality rate for most of these is less than 1 percent, and the complication rate is also low. I won't quibble if my surgical colleagues contend that these are major procedures; they often become so when unexpected difficulties arise.

Both the major and semimajor operations require admission to a hospital and are usually done under general anesthesia, but occasionally spinal anesthetic may be used. None of these should ever be done without complete operating room equipment and personnel.

MINOR SURGERY   Last are the minor operations. There is an incumbent danger in describing any operation as minor, as we shall see. It is seldom considered minor by the patient. Nevertheless, operations of short duration and of a non-life-threatening nature are included in this group. They are often done as short-stay or outpatient procedures for which the patient has only a one- or two-day period of hospitalization or none at all. Some are done in surgical clinics or in doctors' offices. Among the so-called minor operations are breast biopsies, the removal of lumps or cysts, a D & C (dilatation and curettage of the uterus), and perhaps a tonsillectomy. There are many others in this category.

Because the operation is often considered minor by the surgeon, many of these procedures are performed by the marginally qualified (interns and residents) or by those without surgical training at all. Some minor operations may quickly become semimajor procedures. The excision of a lump in the neck, for example, may result in an inadvertent injury to the phrenic nerve to the diaphragm or to the underlying pleura of the lung, with resultant pneumothorax and lung collapse. There are many malpractice suits following less than desirable results from minor surgery. Consider the following example from the report of the Canadian Medical Protective Association of 1975.

A healthy, stocky, moderately obese, 32-year-old father of three children arrived at the hospital at 4 PM where, as an out-patient, he was scheduled to have bilateral excision of deformed and in-grown toe-nails. Previously he had received instructions from the surgeon about

14 The announcement

restricting oral intake to a fluid breakfast but when questioned at the hospital he admitted having had coffee, not only at breakfast, but as late as 12:30 PM. The operation, which had been booked for 5 PM, therefore was deferred until 6 o'clock by which time the anaesthetist who had seen the patient was unavailable and another arrived to give the anaesthetic. This anaesthetist did not question the patient about fluids taken. The man had been mildly reprimanded previously for failing to follow instructions and the reason for the earlier cancellation was recorded on the hospital chart. Intravenous anaesthetic was used and the patient was ventilated with oxygen by mask using an oropharyngeal airway. Because of its anterior location, the larynx could not be visualized and repeated attempts at intubation over a thirty minute period were unsuccessful. Although relaxants were used, on each occasion as their effect wore off, laryngospasm repeatedly occurred and the anaesthetist felt committed to establishing an airway. He called for assistance 15 to 20 minutes after the induction had started and when another anaesthetist arrived ten minutes later he thought he found clinical signs which indicated aspiration had occurred. Ultimately, about 45 minutes after induction, intubation was accomplished by the anaesthetist called to assist. Among the drugs used was Aminophylline, administered intravenously by this anaesthetist on two occasions. A short time after intubation, the patient suddenly became cyanosed and an hour after the anaesthetic had started, suffered a cardiac arrest from which he did not recover. At autopsy the bronchial mucosa appeared swollen and reddened. The pathological diagnosis was haemorrhagic pulmonary oedema, probable aspiration.

At an inquest and subsequent trial it was learned from the patient's widow that the deceased had also taken coffee three hours later than had been previously admitted. The action against the anaesthetists was therefore dismissed. [Pp. 18–20]

Here the results from minor surgery were tragic—following a toenail operation, no less.

Another example of minor surgery resulting in major complications is the following case from the report of the Canadian Medical Protective Association (C. M. P. A.) for 1976.

A middle-aged day labourer was referred for surgical consultation because of a lump on the inner aspect of the lower third of his right arm, present for about a year and said to be enlarging. The surgeon recommended surgical treatment and the man was admitted to hospital. A general physical examination disclosed no abnormalities and, in particular, there were no enlarged lymph nodes. The pre-operative medical record, apparently prepared by a resident, described the lump as round, hard, not painful and about 2 cm. in diameter. There was no mention of its mobility. There were no neurological symptoms and a neurological examination was not carried out. Routine urine examination, haematological examination and biochemical blood studies all were normal as was a chest x-ray. The surgeon confirmed that excision of the mass was indicated and he carried out the surgery under general anaesthesia with tourniquet control. The pre-operative diagnosis was recorded as "tumour lesion of right arm." Although the operative report was brief, it indicated that the surgeon encountered what he thought was a tumour or cyst possibly located in the coracobrachialis tendon. The lesion was resected and the fibrous "structure" with which it was closely associated was joined end to end using black silk sutures. Post-operatively there was a major motor and sensory deficit in the median nerve distribution.

16 The announcement

The precise nature of the tumour was in some doubt for a time but later the pathologist reported it to be a degenerating Schwannoma. Although further surgery for nerve suture was later contemplated, it was never undertaken.

In spite of extensive and prolonged physiotherapy and attempts at rehabilitation, a significant permanent disability prevented the patient from returning to his former employment. When a legal action was brought and the treatment was carefully reviewed, expert opinions could not be obtained in support of the surgeon. It was clear that a lesion involving a nerve had not been recognized as such; there had been no calculated decision about the removal of a portion of median nerve and its inadvertent excision was thought impossible to justify. A substantial settlement had to be made in recognition of the damage suffered. [Pp. 14–16]

The important message here is quite a simple one. Major complications may arise from minor procedures. Therefore, one should not insist on having a general anesthetic for a minor procedure unless it is absolutely indicated or strongly advised by one's surgeon or anesthesiologist. I have performed countless ingrown toenail operations, none of which were done under general anesthetic. It simply is unnecessary most of the time.

The problem with minor operations is simply that—because they are considered minor, they are often given less thoughtful consideration than they merit, even by experienced, well-trained surgeons. Both of the foregoing case reports are examples of unnecessary tragedies. Whether the operation is urgent or elective, major or minor, there are certain things that both patient and surgeon can do to avoid medical or medicolegal disasters.

2 The diagnosis

Since one has little or no choice of surgeon or hospital in the emergency situation, and may have no opportunity to review the diagnosis or to provide informed consent, my remarks are confined to the other categories of operations—those in which one does have an opportunity to review both the diagnosis and the need for surgery.

ESTABLISHING THE DIAGNOSIS

In the matter of diagnosis, there are a number of questions one might and should ask—either of oneself or of the surgeon.

1. *Has the diagnosis been clearly established to one's satisfaction?*
2. *If there are doubts, should a second opinion, another consultation, be obtained?*

Let me point out that a diagnosis, like a weather forecast, is not always certain. Often it is nothing more than an intelligent guess based on surgical judgment founded on the weight of evidence, and sometimes partly based on intuition. Intuition may not be a satisfactory criterion, though, for all patients preparing to undergo an operation.

Nor is a positive diagnosis always possible. Often we must rely on X rays, which have an inherent diagnostic error of anywhere from 15 to 25 percent, depending on the skill of the radiologist rather than on the quality of the X rays. For example, an ulcer may look benign by X ray, yet prove to be malignant at operation. There is always that inevitable margin of error. A CAT (computerized axial tomography) scan may show a mass somewhere in the body, but it doesn't tell us any more about the nature of the mass than whether it is solid (possibly tumor) or cystic (possibly benign).

In some instances establishing a diagnosis may be difficult and take time. A common problem is the patient with anemia. The following case from the C. M. P. A. report of 1975 illustrates some of the problems.

A patient was found to have anemia by his family doctor. The doctor wisely checked his stools for blood and the test was positive. Next, the physician correctly ordered x-rays of the entire gastro-intestinal tract, a barium swallow for the stomach and small bowel, a barium enema for the lower bowel (the colon). The x-rays were negative. An examination of the lower rectum and colon by means of a sigmoidoscope was also clear. The patient was given iron medication and advised to return at a suitable interval. He failed to keep his appointment. His anemia worsened and when he did return, a year later, the x-rays were repeated. This time they disclosed a tumour of the cecum, an area of the large bowel near the appendix in which it is particularly difficult to exclude small tumours by x-ray. At operation, the tumour had spread to involve the liver. A legal action was

> *brought against the family doctor. It was my opinion that the physician could not be held negligent, as he had done everything at the time prescribed by accepted standards of care. The patient was rather more at fault for not having returned for follow-up at the suggested appointment. The action was not pursued in court.*
>
> *A doctor's error of judgment in diagnosis must of itself never be misinterpreted as negligence. A wrong diagnosis or failure of treatment may be considered negligent only if the doctor has failed to meet a reasonable standard of care and competence.*

It is sometimes impossible to avoid delay in diagnosis. It may be tragic when the delay results in an irremediable situation. Sometimes the delay is the fault of the physician or surgeon rather than the patient.

In the C. M. P. A. report of 1975 appears the following case:

> *A forty-six-year-old man visited a family physician's office one morning complaining of tightness in his chest, heartburn and "eructations" of burning fluid into the back of his throat. These symptoms had onset two days earlier. He gave a history of having had a duodenal ulcer in the past. The doctor prescribed an ulcer diet along with anticholinergic tablets and an antacid. He planned to arrange for barium x-ray studies in a day or two. The provisional diagnosis was duodenal ulcer with pylorospasm. Twenty-four hours later when the man reported to the hospital emergency department complaining of abdominal pain, he was seen by a nurse who said he looked pale and was sweating. When informed of this by telephone the doctor ordered an intramuscular injection of Meperidine (for pain) and Promazine Hydrochloride (a tranquilizer). Later in the*

20 The diagnosis

> *day, when informed about persisting symptoms, again by telephone the doctor ordered an ice pack to the abdomen. By 8 o'clock in the evening, on the insistence of the patient's family, he was admitted to hospital where the nurses' notes indicated he was very short of breath with abdominal pain on inspiration; he was bleeding profusely and his pulse was 128 per minute. The doctor did not visit the patient but orders were given for analgesics. The patient received Meperidine Hydrochloride 75 mg. twice during the evening. At 2:30 AM the following morning the nurses found the patient's respirations to be laboured at 48 per minute; there was no palpable radial pulse and apex rate was 156; the doctor was called. He came to examine his patient, the first time since the office visit nearly 40 hours earlier. Blood pressure was then recorded at 100 systolic and the abdominal findings were unremarkable. No additional orders were written and the doctor left. The patient became increasingly restless and confused and died shortly after 6 AM. Autopsy showed a one centimetre perforation of a chronic prepyloric ulcer; the findings suggested to the pathologist a fairly recent perforation of possibly 12 to 24 hours duration. When a legal action was brought and when all the clinical details became known, expert opinions could not support the doctor's work. It was decided a successful defence was impossible and settlement had to be made. [Pp. 16–17]*

Not only was there delay in the diagnosis of perforation, which alone might not have been considered negligent, but there was evidence of improper medical care, which resulted in the successful action against the doctor.

Another example of a delay in diagnosis that resulted in tragedy is the following from the C. M. P. A. report of 1976:

The diagnosis

A 49-year-old woman consulted her doctor, a family physician, with complaints of dizziness, difficulty in focusing her eyes and severe headaches of two week duration. On physical examination the significant finding was a markedly elevated blood pressure of 260/120. Neurological examination was negative. The doctor diagnosed acute hypertensive encephalopathy and admitted the patient to hospital on a Wednesday for investigation and treatment. By Thursday evening after treatment with bed rest and analgesics the blood pressure was lowered to 190/90. On Friday morning the attending doctor requested a consultation by an internist from another town who visited the community regularly twice weekly. Later in the afternoon, although the patient's severe headache was persisting and she had started to vomit, the attending doctor found the physical findings unchanged from the previous day. In particular, a careful funduscopic examination (of the eyes) showed no papilloedema (evidence of increased brain pressure) and after discussing the case by telephone with the consultant who had not yet seen the woman, it was decided to carry out a lumbar puncture. The cerebral spinal fluid pressure was high, over 300 millimetres [normal = 100–200 mm]. The consultant saw the patient a few hours later, early Friday evening. He wrote no note but dictated a consultation report to be typed on Monday. He did not call the attending doctor to discuss the case. In the report which he had dictated but which was not available to the referring doctor, the consultant commented on a history of head injury a month earlier, a history which had not been elicited by the family doctor. He speculated about subdural haematoma as a possible diagnosis and recommended the patient be transferred for a neurological investigation. The following morning, a Saturday, before leaving for

22 The diagnosis

the weekend the family physician saw the patient, found her condition essentially unchanged and assigned her care to a confrere. When the covering physician was called to see the patient Saturday evening, she was drowsy and vomiting; there was of course on the chart no written history, consultation note or progress note to indicate the conclusions which might have assisted in clinical assessment at that time. Late Sunday afternoon when the attending doctor returned and found the patient drowsy, confused and with unequal pupils, he called the consultant. For the first time since the consultant's examination the two doctors compared their findings and concluded the patient should be transferred to the care of a neurosurgeon as soon as possible. The transportation could not be arranged until the following morning but then the patient was transferred to an urban centre where a massive subdural haematoma was evacuated. Although the patient recovered infarction of the visual cortex of the right occipital lobe resulted in a significant field defect on the left and, as well, because of further brain damage the patient was said to have suffered a personality change with emotional instability, intermittent confusion and memory loss. It was the expressed opinion that much or all of the harm could have been prevented by earlier treatment.

When a legal action was brought naming the family doctor, the suit could not be successfully defended and the Court awarded substantial damages for the injuries suffered. [Pp. 18–19]

Here the delay in diagnosis was the result of a serious breakdown in communications between two doctors.

We are all human and we make honest errors; when should a doctor whose error results in delay in diagnosis or incorrect diagnosis be held accountable? In the following case, I'll let you be the judge.

A forty-five-year-old doctor, the father of eight children, underwent open-heart surgery for coronary artery disease, which had been established by X rays (coronary angiograms). The need for surgery was agreed upon. The preliminary workup was complete and included all the required tests and a chest X ray. All went well during and following the operation. There were many X rays taken of the chest in the postoperative period, all of which were reported clear. The patient was discharged.

Two months later, while visiting relatives in a small community, he developed pain in his chest; X rays taken at the community hospital were reported negative. Four months later, because of persistent pain on the same side, another X ray was ordered. On this occasion a lesion or shadow was detected on the opposite side of the chest. A review of all the X rays then revealed that it was present on the preoperative films taken four months previously, as well as on those done in the community hospital.

Another major operation was indicated. The lesion was found to be a tumor, a lung cancer that had spread to at least one lymph node! A lobectomy was performed.

The patient, himself a doctor, was naturally aware of the missed diagnosis. Had the lung tumor been diagnosed first, would he have consented to the open-heart operation? Would he have reversed the order of the operations and had the tumor operation first, since time is of the essence in cancer? If so, would he have been able to withstand it, considering the state of his coronary arteries? Did the stress of the open-heart operation cause increased growth of the tumor? In short, was the patient justified in pursuing legal action? If so, should the first radiologist have been sued? Should those who reported the postoperative films be sued as well, and the radiologist at the community hospital too? What would your decision be if you were the judge? I think that because the lesion on the original film was difficult to detect and could only be seen in retrospect (i.e., after the event), no action should have been undertaken. The interpretation of X rays, as I have stated, is imperfect. Unfortunate, but true. Since the tumor was my own, I made the decision not to pursue the matter further.

A delay in the diagnosis of cancer can have unfortunate consequences. It may result in a shortened prognosis for the patient and may lead to a successful negligence action.

Recently, I was asked by a legal firm to give an opinion in the following case. A forty-five-year-old woman with large, pendulous breasts consulted a plastic surgeon regarding a reduction mammoplasty. The surgeon discovered a small lump in the left breast and, without ordering a mammogram (X rays), elected to perform a bilateral mammoplasty, reasoning that the lump would be removed along with the excess breast tissue. The operative report made no mention of a lump. The presence of the lump in the breast tissue submitted to the hospital pathologist was not recorded on the pathology requisition. Though the breast tissue was sectioned and examined according to established routines, the "lump" was not discovered by the pathologist. His report noted "fibrocystic disease" and "suspicious changes in the ducts of the breast," but no evidence of cancer.

By a mysterious coincidence and under unusual circumstances, the breast tissue was reexamined approximately ten months later, ostensibly for teaching purposes, at which time a cancer of the breast was discovered. The surgeon was notified of this finding, and ultimately, so too was the patient. She was advised then to have a radical mastectomy. Following the operation, residual cancer was discovered in the remaining breast tissue *and* in the lymph node(s) of the axilla (armpit).

Legal action was undertaken against the first pathologist and the hospital, from which she received a substantial settlement. The surgeon was fortunate to have escaped liability for his failure to document the presence of the lump.

UNCERTAINTY ABOUT THE DIAGNOSIS: THE SECOND OPINION

When your diagnosis has not been clearly established, there are certain questions you should ask yourself. Has a thorough workup been done? Such a workup should include a complete history and physical examination, a number of blood tests, and perhaps some X rays prior to admission to the hospital. Will more tests and X rays be done after admission and before your operation? These may well be indicated.

When there is reasonable doubt about the certainty of the diagnosis, one might well ask: "Will I require a second opinion, another consultation?" This may be required for your own protection. In someone with a prior history of heart disease, a consultation with a cardiologist may be necessary to establish your fitness to withstand the operation. If one has chronic lung disease, a consultation with a chest physician may be necessary. Pulmonary function tests may be indicated to determine your ability to undergo a long period of anesthesia. Postponement of your operation may be required for a short time to clear up some preexisting condition—a skin infection, for example—that might represent a hazard to you.

The American College of Surgeons has suggested that second opinions are highly desirable whenever there is doubt about the diagnosis or the need for surgery. In one study it was found that the volume of unnecessary surgery declined significantly whenever second opinions were obtained. What might appear as an absolute indication for surgery to one surgeon would not necessarily be so to a second.

In the United States there is a growing trend toward mandatory second opinions before elective surgery. A report in the *Annals of Surgery* is worth review.* It concerns a study done in relation to second opinions for elective operations. It is called the Cornell Elective Surgery Second Opinion Program, and it involved 7,053 patients who were evaluated for proposed elective surgery between the years 1972 (February) and 1978 (January). The program utilized consultation with a board-certified surgeon for evaluation of the necessity of the recommended elective surgical procedure as the next appropriate therapeutic step.

There were two divisions of second opinion within the program—voluntary and mandatory—depending on the individual unions (or the agency for the second-party payment) involved. In the first such division, a patient recommended for surgery voluntarily scheduled a second opinion through the sponsoring agency. In the second division, the mandatory one, the patient had to obtain a second opinion relevant to the need for surgery in order to receive benefits (i.e., payment of hospital and surgical costs).

The findings of the study are quite startling and also

---

*William R. Grafe, M.D., Charles K. McSherry, M.D., Madelon L. Finkel, M.P.A., and Eugene G. McCarthy, M.D., M.P.H., "The Elective Surgery Second Opinion Program," *Annals of Surgery,* September 1978, *188,* (3), pp. 323–330.

illuminating. Of the total of 7,053 patients, their proposed operations were not confirmed by a board-certified consultant in 27.6 percent of the cases, or approximately 1,946 patients. In other words, between the first and second surgeons, disagreement occurred in more than one out of every four proposed operations!

When the data were broken down according to specialty, orthopedic surgery and gynecologic surgery headed the list of nonconfirmations: Forty-five percent and 31 percent for the voluntary and mandatory divisions were not confirmed by a second orthopedist; and 46 percent and 24.3 percent for the voluntary and mandatory group were not confirmed by a second gynecologist (as shown in the following table). Of the operations proposed, those that were considered unnecessary most frequently by the second consultant were surgery of the knee (48.19 percent), hysterectomies (42.0 percent), prostate operations (41.5 percent), and D & C's (33.3 percent). Surgery of the breast was not confirmed in 28.3 percent of patients, and gallbladder surgery in only 12 percent.

The study also revealed that the rate of nonconfir-

RATE OF CONFIRMATION

Specialty	Voluntary Not Confirmed No.	No.	%	Mandatory Not Confirmed No.	No.	%	Total %
Orthopedics	707	323	45.7	203	63	31.0	42.0
Gynecology	894	358	40.0	522	127	24.3	34.0
Urology	324	117	36.1	158	22	13.9	28.8
Ophthalmology	344	110	32.0	217	45	20.7	27.6
Otolaryngology	491	141	28.7	306	43	14.1	23.0
General Surgery	1375	328	23.9	992	109	11.0	18.0

mation for surgery was higher for non-board-certified surgeons than for those who were certified—though the difference was not considered statistically significant.

The study showed, too, that of the patients followed up for six months to twelve months, 81.8 percent of those who were not confirmed for surgery had not had the surgery performed at a later date. The remainder opted for surgery for a variety of reasons.

What were the reasons for nonconfirmation? These fell into six categories: no pathology shown, medical treatment advised, surgery deferred pending results of medical treatment, surgery approved on an ambulatory basis only, further diagnostic workup considered necessary, and, lastly, surgery contraindicated entirely.

Some examples are as follows: A diagnosis of breast tumor was made in seven patients in whom no lump could be felt; in another an inguinal hernia could not be confirmed; two patients for proposed ulcer surgery had not been tried on medical therapy; an obese female with mildly symptomatic hiatus hernia without reflex was put on a medical regimen and advised to lose weight.

This is not the only study to show similar findings on the matter of second opinion or retrospective review. In Saskatchewan, Canada, between 1970 and 1974 the frequency of hysterectomy decreased by 32.8 percent after a review committee was established to determine the necessity for surgery. This has been called the sentinel effect. The presence of a review committee or the existence of a second opinion program often results in a significant lowering of the frequency of unnecessary operations.

But the American College of Surgeons (ACS) has not stood mutely aside while these developments have transpired. The college presented a critique of these programs in the December 1978 issue of its monthly bulletin. In this report, the claim was made that the savings from the program had been greatly exaggerated—that the cost of ongoing medical treatment and the administrative costs of running the program would largely offset the anticipated savings on surgical and hospital costs in the unconfirmed group of operations. Justifiably, the ACS protests against the use of nonsurgical personnel as second opinion experts, as is the case in some of the programs. It believes strongly that the second opinion should be rendered by a qualified specialist in the appropriate field of surgery.

The college regards the practice of decreasing the payment to a patient who refuses to seek a second opinion as "pernicious." The report further stated: "Mandatory programs that deny or reduce coverage based on a negative second opinion may be construed as interfering with the patient's right to decide on the type and timing of treatment to be received." The ACS's protests may well be too little and too late, however, for it is difficult to argue effectively against the rationale of the program.

So the question of second opinion is important. It may well be that despite the opposition of surgeons, second opinions will become mandatory for all elective operations because the insuring agencies—including Blue Cross, Blue Shield, other insurance companies, and government—will demand it. If one in four or more proposed operations fails to be confirmed by a qualified peer expert, the savings to the insuring agencies may be enormous, to say nothing of the potential saving in lives. Surgeons may have little say in the matter—except to concur.

At St. Michael's Hospital in Toronto, Canada, there has been a dramatic decline over the past ten years in the number of operations for hiatus hernia. This is a hernia of a pouch of stomach through an opening (the hiatus) in the diaphragm. It is usually diagnosed by a barium X ray that discloses the hernia. Some may cause symptoms, others do not; the incidence of such hernias increases with age; they may cause complications in a small percentage of patients, but the complications are rarely fatal. Medical treatment provides relief in many cases, but not a cure. Only surgery can correct the hernia. The operation is a major one and is associated with a definite but low mortality and a moderately high complication rate. And recurrences of the hernia occur in a surprisingly high percentage of patients, 15 to 25 percent in some series.

Because of all these factors, we have performed fewer and fewer hernia operations, in the belief that the surgery is often unnecessary. We have rigidly narrowed our indications for the procedure. However, it is disturbing to learn that the operation is still commonly performed at many other institutions in Ontario Province. Would the frequency of performance decline if a second opinion were sought from an internist or another surgeon? Perhaps not, but the ultimate test might be this: Would the surgeon personally undergo the operation? If surgeons were to apply the same rigid criteria to patients that they would to themselves, it is likely there would be fewer hiatus hernia operations performed.

When the diagnosis is uncertain, it may be advisable for both the patient and the surgeon to have a second opinion or a consultation prior to surgery.

WHEN THE DIAGNOSIS IS CERTAIN

In many instances, the diagnosis will be positively confirmed—for example, by a needle biopsy or an X ray; clearly, there is trouble present. Gallstones are shown on an X ray; a tumor has been diagnosed by a barium enema. Then there is usually no need to review the diagnosis. This can only result in duplication of effort and unnecessary cost—defensive medicine. The patient now asks, what is the need for surgery? In the case of the tumor, both the diagnosis and need are clearly established. Surgery is indicated for a cancer of the bowel; it is better to accept it and get on with it.

However, in the case of a solitary gallstone or a tiny polyp (obviously nonmalignant), the risk of waiting must be balanced against the risk of operation.

If the condition is not causing symptoms, both you and your surgeon may prefer to defer any operation and adopt a watchful policy. In the case of a small inguinal hernia that is causing no trouble, you might wish to wait despite the knowledge that a complication could occur that would require urgent attention later. Usually, a surgeon will advise that the hernia be repaired at once to avoid the likelihood of complication. He or she might, on the other hand, pressure you into an operation by magnifying the dangers. This can be risky; consider the following case:

A forty-six-year-old lawyer noted a mild pain in his groin. He consulted a surgeon who was a personal acquaintance. The surgeon performed a cursory examination and diagnosed a small inguinal hernia. He advised immediate admission to the hospital for repair of the hernia. Before the week was out, this had been arranged. There was no difficulty at the operation. The day following surgery, the patient noted a marked swelling of his testicle and was in extreme pain. Strong narcotics had to be given. The swelling, not uncommon following hernia repairs, did not subside. A fever developed, and antibiotics were given for a presumed infection. Later, the wound showed signs of definite infection. The patient was discharged in spite of the persistent pain and swelling of the testicle. At home, the patient's fever became worse, and redness developed over the testicle. The skin was hot, "like an abscess or boil." The patient was seen at the surgeon's office and was reassured that there was only a little swelling. Subsequently the skin broke down, a large quantity of pus escaped, and the testicle sloughed away. Recovery from the infection was slow, and there was ultimate loss of

> *the testicle, considerable deformity, and persistent pain, especially with intercourse.*

It is my opinion that the surgeon will have difficulty in defending himself against charges of negligence (and possibly malpractice) being brought against him by the lawyer. Both might wonder, too, if the operation was necessary or urgent.

Though complications from repair of inguinal hernia are most unusual, they may occur, especially when there is some doubt about the diagnosis or the need for repair. From the C. M. P. A. report of 1972:

> *A 28-year-old postgraduate student was referred to a surgeon for investigation and treatment of right lower quadrant pain of two to three years' duration. On examination a right indirect inguinal hernia was discovered and this was thought to be the most likely cause of symptoms, although on admission to hospital the same day there was recorded a provisional diagnosis of chronic appendicitis with acute exacerbation. The patient was told his appendix would be removed through the incision used for repair of the hernia. Through a muscle-splitting incision in the right lower quadrant a retrocaecal appendix was located and removed. The posterior wall of inguinal canal was then repaired using what the surgeon described as the McVey technique. No post-operative complications were noted during the four-day post-operative stay in hospital, but ten days after operation the patient returned to the doctor with what were said to be complaints of pain in the right leg, particularly in the calf. There was said to be calf tenderness and the diagnosis of thrombophlebitis was made and treatment recommended. Subsequently the patient consulted another surgeon who found weakness of the thigh and sensory loss, all diagnostic of a*

femoral nerve lesion. Following appropriate neurological examination, observation and physiotherapy over a five-month period during which there was no improvement in the symptoms, the femoral nerve was explored and extensive scarring and neuroma formation was found involving the nerve at a point well proximal to the inguinal ligament. This area was excised and the nerve trunk sutured. The microscopic description of the excised specimen was as follows: "piece of fibrous tissue containing large oedematous nerve bundles. In the surrounding connective tissue are numerous sutures, foreign body type of granulomas." Although the final result of nerve suture was reasonably satisfactory the patient will likely have some permanent atrophy and weakness of thigh muscles and altered skin sensation over the right knee and calf. When a legal action was brought and when all the clinical details were known it became obvious the doctor could not be defended. Although the precise manner in which the femoral nerve was injured was never explained the neuroma with adjacent suture material and foreign body reaction so strongly implicated the surgeon that a settlement had to be made. [Pp. 21–22]

It would seem vital, then, if you are to have an operation and wish to avoid a potential disaster, that you choose your surgeon carefully.

3 How to pick your surgeon

No doctor would be so naive as to assume that all surgeons are of equal ability; nor should a patient. Just as artists are of different caliber (and command different fees for their work), so too are surgeons. There are many varieties of surgeons, and it is of value to explain what each does.

General surgeons perform a broad spectrum of operations, from hernias to varicose veins to breast operations. They may, if trained in these subspecialties, do some plastic procedures, urological operations, orthopedic work, even chest surgery. For the most part today, especially in larger centers, the general surgeon has become essentially a gastrointestinal surgeon. He or she may or may not handle trauma—accidents, gunshot wounds, and the like.

The orthopedic surgeon deals with fractures and diseases of the bones and joints; a plastic surgeon treats burns and does reconstructive and cosmetic operations; a urologic surgeon manages conditions of the kidney, ureter, bladder, and prostate gland; neurosurgeons confine themselves to abnormalities of the brain, spinal cord, and peripheral nerves; a gynecologist specializes in diseases of the female genital tract—uterus, fallopian tubes and ovaries, cervix, vagina—but often combines this with obstetrics. An opthalmologist performs operations on the eye, and an otolaryngologist specializes in problems of the ear, nose, throat, and upper respiratory system. At one time these two specialities were combined but seldom are any longer. A pediatric surgeon deals exclusively with children, but he or she may be a pediatric general surgeon, urologist, or neurosurgeon—a specialist within a specialty. Some surgeons specialize in cancer (e.g., at New York Memorial Hospital) and operate on a single organ for the most part (breast service or thoracic service). Cardiac surgeons, of course, operate on the heart but may perform procedures on the aorta or limb vessels as well. In some hospitals these two areas are divided into two specialties. Thoracic surgeons limit themselves primarily to diseases of the lung or esophagus.

CRITERIA

It is logical to ask, do surgeons have different technical abilities from one speciality to another? In a sense they do, since each surgical discipline demands special skills. But I don't believe that one group has greater overall skills than another. Individually, they are all different; as a group, however, I don't believe that plastic surgeons have greater innate skill than neurosurgeons or urologists, for example. The surgeons themselves may believe otherwise, but there is little evidence to substantiate such a belief. Then why does the plastic surgeon charge more for services than the gynecologist? The charge is higher because the paying public believes that the plastic surgeon's services are worth more and is willing to pay more for them. Plastic surgery and neurosurgery convey in the public mind an unwarranted image of technical superiority that borders on the realm of magic or fantasy. I believe that surgeons should receive fees that are commensurate with their training, experience, and ability rather than with their specialty or the nature of the operation. Why should an operation on the heart—an A/C [aorto/coronary] bypass, for example—which is becoming exceedingly common, command a greater fee than an operation of equal magnitude for a brain tumor or a cancer of the pancreas? In Canada, for example, there is an inexplicable discrepancy in the fees for these three operations ($654.50 for the bypass, $490 for a craniotomy, $500 for a pancreatectomy). In the United States these figures are paltry by comparison and in most major centers could easily be quadrupled.

The greatest injustice, however, both to patients and surgeons, is that a poorly qualified surgeon may charge as much or more than the highly qualified surgeon! The fee, then, is not a measure of the surgeon's technical competence, whatever you may believe to the contrary, but more about fees later.

QUALIFICATIONS, TRAINING, EXPERIENCE, AND RESULTS In choosing a surgeon, then, one's first concern should be for the qualifications, training, experience, and results of that surgeon and for nothing else. A measure of these indices can be made partly by the surgeon's degrees, which often reflect his or her training.

How then can you tell if your surgeon is qualified? In the United States he or she will have passed the American Board Examinations in surgery (i.e., be board certified) or will be board eligible (i.e., qualified to write the exams). In many instances, the surgeon will also be a Fellow of the American College of Surgeons. Beware if your surgeon is none of these or is self-trained or a general-practitioner (GP) surgeon. The risk one takes in undergoing an operation by an unqualified surgeon is magnified many times over.

Is there any evidence to support this contention? The

Trussell Report of 1964 showed that board-certified surgeons and/or members of the American College of Surgeons provided good or excellent treatment doing major surgery in 66 percent of the instances (48 of 73 cases); the nonspecialists in 51 percent of the cases (18 of 35), and GP surgeons only 20 percent of the time (1 of 5). Admittedly the numbers are small, but they reflect the differences fairly accurately.

In the United States one-third of the surgeon pool is made up of noncertified surgeons and general-practitioner surgeons.* Yet these surgeons performed 32 to 41 percent of the total operations done in four geographical areas within the continental United States in 1970. The reason for the high percentage of unqualified surgeons here is quite simple. The United States is a highly democratic country, and *failure by a surgeon to achieve board certification does not limit one's ability to practice surgery provided that he can obtain hospital privileges.* Surprising indeed!

The reason there are so many surgeons in the United States practicing without board certification may be partly due to the high failure rates of candidates on the examinations. For the American graduates, this averages 14 percent; but for foreign medical graduates, it has averaged 50 percent! The number of noncertified surgeons who are permitted to practice in the United States continues to grow.

But are these not trained surgeons who fail? The tragedy of the matter is that they are; most have spent a minimum of four years in surgical residency programs. Some of the programs are accredited, others are not. Many of the unsuccessful candidates should have been weeded out in the early years of training by a preliminary examination— a mandatory, in-service qualifying exam that would determine a candidate's suitability to complete four years of training.

The quality of training is also important. Some can-

---

*Bulletin of the American College of Surgeons, March 1976.

didates with four years of "training" have served mainly as observers or junior residents, or have held positions of little responsibility. Some have performed few major operations at all. I have examined foreign graduates for the F. R. C. S. (Fellows of the Royal College of Surgeons) exams who have appeared without ever having done some of the most common gastrointestinal operations in general surgery.

But surely, you protest, to be a surgeon, one must have a minimum of technical expertise. Surely surgeons are trained in the animal laboratory, their technical ability screened by an expert surgical teacher; not necessarily so. Rarely are such screening techniques part of surgical training programs. Instruction in the lab on the art of tying ligatures, dissecting, and performing operations is not part of most surgical programs. Then how can the public be protected from stumblebums, those who do not have innate technical skills? Unfortunately, it can't be completely, for as I have pointed out, those who fail their boards can still practice surgery in the United States.

The American College of Surgeons is trying to correct these deficiencies by holding in-service examinations early in surgical programs to allow a candidate to qualify for the boards. It is simply not fair to the public or to the candidates to allow them to finish four years of training if they should have been plucked earlier.

Apart from qualifications and training, the other factors that are important in choosing one's surgeon are experience and results. In this area, there is considerably more difficulty in making an assessment, because experience and results are qualities that cannot be listed along with a surgeon's degrees. In the United States today, doctors are permitted to advertise, but traditional views of ethics and professionalism make it unlikely that the following slogans will soon be common: "Would you rather convalesce in Florida or take out funeral insurance?" "Why have a colostomy when you don't need one?" "Worried about sexual impotence after your operation? We guarantee success."

But experience *is* important. Who would you prefer to do your open-heart operation—a surgeon who has done 1,000 of them or someone embarking on the first ten? Or your gallbladder operation? Would you not prefer a surgeon who has done several hundred to one who does relatively few? Other factors being equal, a surgeon's mortality rates and complication rates improve (i.e., are lowered) with experience, especially for major operations. Experienced surgeons have more confidence; they have overcome the technical problems through practice, trial, and error, and one hopes they have profited from their mistakes.

Recently a thirty-year-old woman underwent what should have been a routine gallbladder operation. There was a suggestion on the X ray of stones in the main bileduct. Exploration of the bile-duct was called for. The surgeon tried a new instrument with which he was not familiar, a fiber-optic visual aid called a choledochoscope, which permits direct visualization of the bile-ducts. Being unfamiliar with it, he pumped air into the ducts (saline is called for) under extreme pressure. The ducts of the liver were ruptured, and air entered the main vessels of the liver. Massive air embolism resulted, and the woman died. Another surgeon, with experience in over 100 of these examinations, reported no complications and no deaths from the same procedure! As we shall see in a later chapter, failure to use equipment properly or to check out equipment in use is increasingly becoming a cause of legal action.

Obviously, the most important part of surgery is the result. Fortunately, the outcome for the majority of procedures done today in the United States is good if not excellent. Mortality rates for the most common procedures, even those of great magnitude (coronary-artery bypass, for example) are below 3 percent. The mortality for major gastric operations is less than 3 percent also; and for gallbladder surgery, it is well under 1 percent. These figures prevail in the larger centers that report their results in surgical journals. There is a wide swing in mortality rates from center to center though. This depends on the surgeon, the hospital or clinic, and the type of patient.

For example, the mortality rates quoted by the Mayo and Lahey Clinics for pancreatectomy, one of the most difficult operations known, is in the neighborhood of 8 to 10 percent. Few centers can match these figures. Why? At these clinics only a few surgeons perform this operation. They have greater experience and greater numbers—in the hundreds. And their patients are usually well-to-do (though not always) and are thus in better general physical condition than patients operated on at the New Orleans Charity Hospital, for example.

So results do vary. Usually, though, a patient does not have access to surgical journals in which results of procedures are reported. How can you find out about a surgeon's results? Quite simply, you may ask your family physician or the clinician who referred you to the surgeon. But this is rarely done.

MAKING AN INTELLIGENT CHOICE

Knowing the importance of the foregoing, let us consider some practical approaches to the task of picking a surgeon. You should ask yourself these questions:

1. *Is he or she qualified? This is something you can find out from your referring doctor or from the surgeon.*

2. *Does the practitioner work at an accredited hospital? This can be learned in the same way—by asking.*

3. *Has your physician ever seen your surgeon operate, actually assisted him or her during an operation?*

Many family physicians assist surgeons during operations on their private patients, but some do not. If your referring doctor has assisted your surgeon and attests to his or her competence, that is the best recommendation there is. If your family doctor does not assist the surgeon, then you can't be as certain.

4. Does your family doctor work out of the same clinic as your surgeon?

This may seem to be of little consequence, but the American College of Surgeons is aware from studies it has done that the incidence of unnecessary surgery is higher among surgeons in group practice than among those in solo practice. Surprised? You shouldn't be. What is an eager young surgeon to do when referred a "gall bladder" or "uterine fibroid" by a close colleague and a member of the same club? Reply that surgery isn't indicated? Refer the patient back for more tests? Get a second opinion? Not very likely. His or her colleague would certainly not refer many more cases in these categories. Besides, in most clinics or group practices, the surgeon is often a partner in the group. In fact, the surgeon is often the most important partner from a financial standpoint, because the highest fees are in the surgical domain; more surgery means more income for the group; more income means a higher share of the profits for other members of the group. The surgeon's fees often carry the clinic; the other members of the clinic therefore have a vested interest in providing the surgeon with cases for surgery.

5. Who does your family doctor go to for surgical operations?

What about surgery for other members of the doctor's family—his or her spouse and children? If you can find this out, you are well ahead of the game. The highest respect a physician can pay a surgeon is to be that surgeon's patient or to send family members to him or her. The greatest accolade is to be called "a doctor's surgeon." You can be certain that "doctor's surgeons" will be good: they will have been thoroughly checked out; they don't do unnecessary surgery; and their mortality rates are low. Physicians have a great advantage over their patients in this regard. For my two operations, both performed in the same hospital where I operate, I had my pick of surgeons. I was lucky. But do you believe for a minute that I would have submitted to either procedure (A/C bypass and lobectomy—both major operations) had I not been certain of my surgeon's results? After all, the Cleveland Clinic is but a short hop by air from Toronto. There, the results of A/C bypass are slightly lower than for any other center in the United States. I knew this, but I also knew that the results at our hospital were just about as good.

Consider the opposite situation—a small facility in Massachusetts. In a small suburban hospital there, a group of surgeons is being investigated by state health officials because of an extremely high death rate among patients undergoing open-heart surgery. The mortality rate was reported to be 33 deaths out of 64 patients, ten times that of leading centers. Where would you prefer to have your open-heart operation—at the small suburban hospital or at the Cleveland Clinic?

Dr. William A. Nolen, author of *Surgeon Under the Knife,* describes in detail how he chose the surgeon for his own A/C bypass.* Of course, he did a lot of research, too; in fact he was doing it for an article for *Esquire* magazine when he discovered that he needed an A/C bypass himself. Being a surgeon, Dr. Nolen wasn't about to let a beginner

---

*William A. Nolen, *Surgeon Under the Knife* (New York: Dell Publishing Co., Inc., 1977).

practice on him. Of course, facilities were not present in the community hospital in Litchfield, Minnesota, where he operated, but they were available in Minneapolis and in Rochester, Minnesota. But Dr. Nolen was not satisfied with the preoperative attention he received at the hospital of his first choice. He criticized (rather unfairly, I thought) the cardiologist for not having reviewed some of his tests sooner. Dr. Nolen believed that a delay of six days before reading an electrocardiogram was intolerable. He considered the Houston and the Mayo Clinics ("too cold and impersonal"), the Cleveland Clinic ("an academic upheaval" was going on), and finally chose the Massachusetts General Hospital in Boston on the advice of a medical friend.

Dr. Nolen checked out three surgical clinics in the country before deciding on a fourth, out of state. He even rejected the Mayo Clinic in Rochester, Minnesota, within driving distance of his home. Why shouldn't you make similar decisions?

This raises another question. Does your own doctor leave the community for surgical operations? You can appreciate that when the magnitude of the operation is similar to that of an A/C bypass, and when facilities are not available locally for the procedure, one has no choice but to go elsewhere. But for a semimajor or minor procedure, does your doctor have the local surgeon perform it or go elsewhere? Is an outside surgeon brought in? What is good enough for patients coming to the clinic may not be good enough for the doctor!

6. *Does your surgeon have an obvious physical or mental handicap?*

I have known surgeons to continue to operate when they were severely myopic, were senile, had tremors from neurological disease, were obviously alcoholic, or were even psychotic. Yet they were allowed to continue to practice.

When I first started practice as a GP in a small community in Northern Ontario, the chief surgeons of two hospitals were chronic alcoholics. The doctors all knew it, and so did many of their patients. Some mornings, the smell of alcohol from the surgeon's breath was so strong coming across the OR table that his assistants nearly passed out.

But a myopic surgeon operating? Yes, indeed! A man from Toronto chose as his surgeon one whose vision was terribly impaired. The operation was in the semimajor category—a cholecystectomy. The surgeon completely divided the common bile-duct—even after he had been warned by his assistant—and a disaster occurred. The patient developed a fistula, became jaundiced, and died after an unsuccessful attempt by a second surgeon to repair the damage.

Another surgeon with whom I worked in my early days of training was mentally unstable. I once walked out on him during an operation and told him I'd never assist him again. He deserved the unkind sobriquet of butcher. Many of his patients died because of his incompetence. Fortunately, this type of surgeon is rare today. For the most part, those with physical handicaps do not go into surgery, because it demands a degree of physical fitness unrequired of other specialties. There seems to be a process of natural selection of the species at work.

7. *Are you certain that your surgeon will actually perform the operation personally?*

In the majority of instances, one can reasonably expect that this will be the case, but not always. In the United States today, "ghost" surgeons are rare. What are "ghost" surgeons? Like ghosts, they steal in unseen by the patient and depart after the operation—with a portion of the surgical fee. The patient may never know that the "ghost" performed the operation. The "ghost" is brought in by your GP or by the surgeon you expected to do the operation. Ghost surgery is unethical because two principles of trust are broken: first, you have not consented to the ghost surgeon; and second, there has been fee splitting—part to the GP, part to "your" surgeon, and part to the ghost surgeon.

In some instances the ghost surgeon is in fact a resident surgeon in training. How can this be? If a resident is assigned to do an operation in a teaching hospital without any supervision by the attending surgeon, it represents a form of ghost surgery, especially if the fee for the procedure is pocketed by the absentee surgeon. The fee or a part of it may go to the hospital—some for research, some for administration, and some for salaries—but the principle is the same: there has been a division of the fee, and the patient did not get the contracted-for individual as surgeon. In some institutions the consent form will clearly state that your surgeon may choose to assign your operation to a subordinate. This is accepted practice in all teaching institutions; otherwise, how would the surgeons of the future be taught? As long as you are aware of this when you sign your consent form, there has been no breach of contract. Fortunately, ghost surgery is declining in frequency in North America.

SOURCES OF INFORMATION Finally, there are several sources of information that you definitely should *not* rely on when making your choice of surgeon. First of all, a friend or neighbor, no matter how well-meaning, should never be relied on for accuracy, even if that person has had the same operation that you're going to have. They just don't know. Nor should one rely on auxiliary hospital or paramedical personnel, such as a physiotherapist, X-ray technician, orderly, nurse's aid, or nurse. Even a nurse on a surgical floor cannot properly evaluate a surgeon's competence unless he or she has been head nurse for a number of years and knows who has the greatest number of complications and who does not. They have their favorites among the surgical staff, but the choice is usually based on the surgeon's attitude toward them rather than on technical ability.

Surgical scrub nurses may not be as wise in their choice of surgeon as one might think. They are close to the surgeon, it is true; but they are less impressed with what he is doing than with how quickly it is done, and with whether the doctor is affable toward them and pleasant to work with. They seldom see the postoperative complications.

One morning in the operating room at St. Michael's Hospital, I was presented with a new scrub nurse. She had worked in the OR of a small community hospital in Ontario where I knew all the surgeons well. I asked her if she had worked with them and who she thought was the best. Her choice of surgeon left me speechless, since this surgeon regularly referred a string of incredible complications to our hospital, most of which were the result of his mismanagement.

The only person whom one can rely on who does work at the hospital is the surgical intern or resident—the person who, in a teaching institution, usually assists or is assisted by your prospective surgeon. The resident works with the surgeon every day, checks diagnoses and preoperative workups, sees him or her perform operations of every magnitude, and checks the patients following those operations. If a resident says that a surgeon is good, 99 percent of the time you can be certain of the accuracy of the statement.

But what if there are no teaching hospitals in your community? And what if there are, but you are not acquainted with any of the residents? Then you must find out from your family physician. He or she will be reliable most of the time.

One GP, when asked how he picked a surgeon for his patients, said that he used a "Three-*A*" system: *A* for availability (for his and the patient's convenience), *A* for affability (toward both him and his patient), and, last, *A* for ability. Though he probably had them in reverse order of importance, at least he included ability. You should, too!

There are some things that you would have trouble finding out about your surgeon that could have a bearing on your future relationship—especially if you were unhappy later with the result. It would be of value to know whether your surgeon is litigation prone—if he or she has been sued more than once (one in four are eventually) and, if so, whether successfully or not. It would be helpful to learn if this individual gets along well with his or her colleagues or is considered a renegade. You would be interested, naturally, to learn if your prospective surgeon is in good standing with the local surgical or medical society, if his or her license has ever been under suspension, if he or she has ever been in trouble with the law because of drugs, drunken driving, or other criminal offenses. It would also be of value to know whether your surgeon keeps up with the most recent scientific advances, attends surgical meetings, takes self-assessment exams (SESAP—Surgical Education and Self-Assessment Program of the American College of Surgeons), agrees to peer review by superiors or to recertification review.

I'm afraid that not even a private detective could uncover all these things. And besides, to permit one to do so would be a grave infringement on personal liberty. But if you did know, it might make a considerable difference in your choice of surgeon, might it not?

4 Choosing your hospital

Choosing your hospital is only slightly less important than choosing your surgeon. For the most part, the standard of a hospital is a reflection of the standard of its surgical (and medical) staff. Good hospitals tend to have good surgeons, and vice versa. The previously mentioned Trussell report noted a wide divergence of results following major surgery when teaching hospitals were compared with voluntary, proprietary, and municipal hospitals. Teaching hospitals were judged 92 percent "eminently successful" as against 55 percent for their counterparts. Generally, the noncertified and GP surgeons practiced in the smaller voluntary, proprietary, and community hospitals. Another study conducted by the Health Information Foundation revealed that in hospitals under 50 beds, 80 percent of surgery was performed by nonspecialists, and mainly by GPs (65 percent) in hospitals under 100 beds. In hospitals in the 100 to 250 range, by contrast, nearly 60 percent of the surgery was performed by specialists, and in those over 500 beds, 80 percent. Size of hospital, then, generally reflects both the percentage of qualified surgeons on staff and the quality of surgery performed.

PEOPLE AND MACHINES MATTER

The reason for the differences in the quality of care in various institutions has to do partly with the facilities available in the institution and partly with the caliber of the paramedical staff—nurses, technicians, orderlies, and so forth. Obviously, it is difficult to provide first-rate surgical care in second-rate institutions—hospitals without proper equipment.

In a small proprietary institution in Toronto, an operation was performed under general anesthesia, and cardiac arrest occurred. There was no equipment in the operating room for cardiac resuscitation. The outcome was foreordained.

In the United States, there is a wide variety of hospital facilities. They include such highly prestigious institutions as the Mayo Clinic, the Lahey Clinic, Massachusetts General, and the Ochsner Clinic; hospitals that specialize in particular patient populations, such as children's and veterans' hospitals; facilities that limit themselves in the type of health care administered there, such as maternity hospitals, cancer treatment centers, and psychiatric hospitals. There are teaching hospitals that are affiliated with medical schools and serve as the beneficiaries (and guinea pigs) of some of the work being done in those research centers. And, of course, there are myriad small, private hospitals and federal, state, county, and municipal facilities all over the country.

Medical and hospital care in the United States is diverse in quality, cost, and accessibility. The level of expertise in diagnosis and treatment is, in some instances, the best in the world. The costs, however, are sometimes prohibitive to many. National health care, not yet instituted, is a tangle of legislative controversy. Lawmakers battle over whether it should become a reality at all, what it should cover, and how it should be financed.

Although there is Medicare (for older citizens) and Medicaid (for the medically indigent), not all eventualities are covered. Many people do have medical and surgical insurance coverage through Blue Cross and Blue Shield (as well as other medical insurers), either privately or through group plans partially or totally funded by their employers. What is termed a "catastrophic illness," however, can still destroy a family's monetary assets in a relatively short period of time, because coverage is limited.

Costs for labor and technology have risen to such levels in the United States that there are extant facilities being closed because the money to pay people to operate the equipment is simply not available. This is particularly true with city facilities (e.g., in New York City), which are funded from already strapped municipal budgets. Strikes for higher wages and better working conditions by aides and technicians, nurses, and even by interns and residents are not uncommon. Such strikes are, of course, made more likely by the soaring rate of inflation in the country.

Choosing your hospital, then, can be a matter of life and death, nearly as important as choosing your surgeon; for as we have seen, the two are often interrelated. So many things can go wrong that the list of disasters is endless. Just being in a hospital can be dangerous to your health; and this is aside from the problems that may arise in the operating theater. What are some of the things that can go wrong that may lead to medicolegal action?

HOSPITAL HAZARDS

First there is the matter of medications. This is one of the most common areas of human error. Medication may be given to the wrong patient; to the correct patient, but in the wrong dose; or by the wrong route—intramuscular instead of by mouth. They may be administered over too long a period (someone forgot to discontinue them), or there may be failure to administer them altogether. Accidents may occur during their administration—by injection, for example—and are a never-ending source of difficulty. Antibiotics are especially prone to cause problems because of their toxic side effects and the possibility of patients developing allergic reactions to them.

In California, a study of potentially compensable events revealed that *nosocomial* infections (i.e., those acquired in the hospital) caused 29.3 percent of injuries that could lead to liability. Antibiotics and other drugs caused 11 percent of the injuries; so the surgeon or physician was doubly liable in 40 percent of the injuries—first, for the infection; and second, for damage caused by the antibiotic used to combat the patient's infection.

Just being in a hospital bed can be a potential problem—for both patient and doctor. A study by the National Association of Insurance Commissioners disclosed that in a one-year period, 25 percent of malpractice claims resulted from the patient falling, usually out of bed. Of course many of these and other falls occur in patients who are infirm.

The list of human errors is endless, but some of them are worth enumerating. Broken thermometers and enema tips; burns from hot sitz baths and hot water bottles; disappearing drains; and broken IV catheters, bladder catheters, and other internal devices may result in complications and personal injury claims. Other areas of potential problems noted in the California study that were outside the operating room were in the radiotherapy and radiology departments.

So even without surgery, accidents may occur just from being in the hospital. It is necessary then to choose your hospital carefully. Here are some questions that you should ask yourself, your doctor, or your surgeon.

Is the hospital accredited? Remember that if it is not, the caliber of surgery may not be high. Uncertified surgeons may perform the bulk of the surgery.

In the United States, the Joint Commission on Accreditation of Hospitals (JCAH) periodically investigates hospital facilities and their administration to decide whether an institution may be accredited. Once achieved, the standards of accreditation must be maintained, and the JCAH can retract a hospital's standing if they are not. Government aid to a hospital may be withdrawn if accreditation is lost. The JCAH is made up of representatives of a number of organizations, including the American Medical Association, the American College of Surgeons, and the American Hospital Association.

What is the bed capacity of the hospital? If under fifty beds, as we have noted, there may be less than adequate facilities and a less than adequately trained staff. Certainly we all know of small clinics with a bed capacity under fifty where excellent work is done. The Shouldice Clinic in Toronto, Canada, which specializes in the repair of hernias, is an example of such an institution. It has an excellent local and international reputation. Many of its patients are referred by doctors in the United States. Its rate of hernia recurrence is one of the lowest in the world. It is an exception to the rule.

One should anticipate, too, when entering a small private hospital, that the rates for any operation may be higher than for hospitals in the intermediate category. Though the larger teaching hospitals would seem to present less risk because of the higher percentage of certified surgeons on their staffs, one must remember, too, that although the fee may be lower, there is a greater likelihood that residents in training will participate in, or actually perform, one's operation. This is not necessarily a bad thing. If your hospital is duly accredited for surgical training, then the caliber of surgical resident is likely to be high. This has presented a problem in the United States. To carry on teaching programs, many nonaccredited hospitals have been forced to accept foreign-trained medical graduates on their programs. The more prestigious the institution, the less difficulty it has in attracting outstanding candidates for surgical training.

Permit me one demonstration of pride and satisfaction. St. Michael's Hospital in Toronto, which is affiliated with the University of Toronto postgraduate surgical training program, and where I have been an attending surgeon, has for years attracted superior surgical residents. The source of my pride in our hospital and its surgical program is that year after year, it has been listed as the first choice for training by the greatest number of applicants of any of the five or six major teaching hospitals in Toronto. We literally have our pick of residents for the general surgery department.

Is the staff of the hospital compatible? This is something that you may never find out about, but occasionally doctors do wash their dirty linen in public. In Pembroke, a small city in Ontario, there was a division of sentiment within the community, pro and con, concerning a surgeon charged by his colleagues with incompetence, mismanagement, and probably other things as well. It could not help but have a deleterious effect on the entire community. The controversy received full-page coverage in the *Toronto Globe* and *Mail*. Whether for good reason or not, a patient simply had to think twice before choosing that surgeon.

In another instance a surgeon in Toronto was refused surgical privileges in a hospital near his office, more than likely because of personality conflicts with other members of the staff. Though the stated reasons given by the board for its refusal were that the hospital had a full complement of surgeons, that the surgeon in question already had another hospital appointment, and that his letters of reference were not impressive, the unstated reason was "that he failed to illustrate—that blend of education, expertise, special skills and character which filled a need." He appealed his case to a higher court of Ontario, and the hospital's position was upheld.* Though there was much sympathy for him outside the hospital and a considerable body of opinion that he was being discriminated against, it would have been an unhappy situation if he had won. The disharmony among the staff and the isolation of the individual would have created an intolerable situation.

The courts in Ontario also upheld the Board of Scarborough General Hospital for dismissing a qualified orthopedic surgeon from its staff because of his "abrasive personality."† The reasons given by the board for his dismissal were that he failed to show "the degree of competence to be expected and has demonstrated that he is abrasive, arrogant and is not amenable to continuing education from his colleagues." Apparently, then, surgeons themselves think enough of the importance of harmony to go so far as to dismiss a colleague. For some illogical reason, though, surgeons are seldom dismissed for genuine incompetence. There seems to be a *laissez-faire* attitude prevailing (widely accepted among members of the surgical club) that if someone is already on the team, he or she should be retained.

Dismissal for incompetence is not only rare but risky. An example is of a urological surgeon, a member of the kidney transplant team, who was dismissed from the Calgary Foothills Hospital in Alberta, Canada.‡ His privileges were revoked "because his presence constituted a disruptive influence in the hospital." There was also "an allegation of

---

*MacDonald and North York General Hospital (1976), 90. R (2d) 143 (H.C.)

†Schiller and Board of Governors of the Scarborough General Hospital (1975). 61 D. L. R. (3d) 416 (Ont. C. A.)

‡Abouna. Foothills Provincial General Hospital Bd. (No. 2) (1978) 83 D. L. R. 333 (Alta. C. A.)

professional misconduct," and "the [transplant team] could not operate in harmony" with him. Perhaps there were other reasons why he was not permitted to operate; one can only surmise. He sued the hospital for $100,000 for loss of his freedom to practice, and he won. This award was later reduced to $10,000 on appeal.

In the United States, according to an article in the *Bulletin of the American College of Surgeons**:

> *Testimony of colleagues, administrative staff, or nursing personnel concerning the physician's inappropriate behavior, as well as documentation of a physician's villification of others, screaming, and use of profanity in the hospital have been considered sufficient to support [in court] a denial or revocation of staff privileges. [P. 22]*

Usually, "where there's smoke there's fire," and one would be well advised to avoid choosing a hospital where politics, rather than patient care, is the main concern of the staff or where disharmony and pettiness prevail. There is often more to the imbroglio than ever reaches the newspapers. Few doctors will openly charge another member of their staff with incompetence, unnecessary surgery, high mortality rates, mismanagement of patients, or reckless lack of concern for a patient's welfare. Such charges are difficult to prove—and they lend themselves to countersuits for defamation of character.

One might ask another question, though the chances of it being answered are slim: Does the hospital provide for the review of the mortality and complication rates? Most large, university, and metropolitan hospitals have at least

---

*Michael E. Reed, JD, with the firm of Vedder, Price, Kaufman and Kammholz, Chicago, "Can Personality Affect Hospital Privileges?" *Bulletin of the American College of Surgeons,* 1980, 65 (4), pp. 19, 22.

a semblance of a tissue committee to maintain their accreditation. These are usually composed of a pathologist along with a member of the departments of surgery and gynecology. The object of the committee is a periodic review of the tissue specimens removed over a specific period of time—the appendixes, gallbladders, and uteri. The purpose of the review, ostensibly, is to serve as a check on the number of normal organs removed; and the three aforementioned organs lead the list—especially the uterus. Hysterectomy is reported to be the most frequently performed and unnecessary operation in North America. The surgical removal of tonsils, appendixes and gallbladders is close behind, but tonsillar tissue is seldom reviewed since it doesn't lend itself to such appraisal—it usually looks normal. If there are too many normal looking appendixes, gallbladders, and uteri, the committee is charged with the duty of drawing this fact to the attention of the offending surgeon(s) or gynecologist(s). The presence of a tissue committee is not an infallible safeguard against unnecessary surgery, however. In a review of five hospitals, Dr. Virgil Stee reported in the *Bulletin of the American College of Surgeons* that the incidence of unnecessary operations varied markedly from hospital to hospital. The percentage of operations that was considered "justified" by an examination of "diseased" tissue varied from a low of 40 percent for hysterectomy at one hospital to a high of 100 percent for cholecystectomy (gallbladder) at another. His findings revealed that overall, 26 percent of the operations involved normal or slightly diseased tissues. And in many operations (hiatus hernia, exploratory laparotomy, vein ligation, uterine suspension) in which a degree of surgical judgment is involved, there is no tissue specimen to examine!

But the tissue committee, in fact, seldom slaps a surgeon on the knuckles and advises restraint. Most tissue committees are without clout, and their record of meetings serves the primary essential purpose of preserving the accreditation of the hospital. They look good in theory and satisfy the inspectors, but in practice they are often impotent.

One might assume that every hospital should be required to review regularly its mortality and complication rate. This is true, but the requirements are poorly spelled out, and some institutions pay only lip service to this rule. The only reference to a mortality review committee (medical or surgical) in the *Guide to Hospital Accreditation* (1977) is contained in a list of the "essential characteristics of an acceptable patient care evaluation procedure."* The final procedural requirement (of a list of six) states: "Documented reports of the results of all audit activities must go to the appropriate clinical departments, the medical advisory committee, the chief of the medical staff and to the hospital's governing body. Included in this audit must be a tissue review, the analysis of deaths and necropsy reports, utilization review, use of consultations, and review of infections and complications."

In Canada, not all hospitals have a standing mortality review committee, and fewer still hold regular meetings—death rounds. At our hospital they were seldom held (regularly), records of them were infrequently kept, and there was rarely (if ever) an audit. The attendance at them, unlike the weekly medical or surgical rounds, was sparse. The single most important conference—the one that should provide the greatest value for avoiding similar mistakes, suggesting improvements in care, and making changes; the one that should offer the greatest learning experience to the staff—is often the most poorly organized and attended. Doctors simply don't like having their mistakes held up for

---

*Guide to Hospital Accreditation (Ottowa, Canadian Council on Accreditation, 1977), pp. 21–23.

review. Surgical grand rounds, on the other hand—where the successes are presented—are far more popular. It's simply human nature, and doctors are, after all, human.

One might well ask, then, if the tissue committee is impotent, how can unnecessary operations be prevented? If no mortality conferences are held, how can one be certain that the same mistake won't happen again—to you? The frequency of unnecessary surgery can be reduced by asking for a second opinion; but this too is seldom done, although medical insurance companies, in particular, are urging patients to get a second opinion more and more often. How can one recognize the surgeon who performs an unacceptably high percentage of unnecessary operations? Let us consider the next step in the process of having an operation—meeting your surgeon.

5 Meeting your surgeon: the verbal contract

Now, if you are satisfied with the diagnosis and the need for surgery, and have made your choice of a surgeon (it is often made for you at this point), and have agreed to be admitted to the hospital of your (doctor's) choice, it is still quite likely that you will not yet have met your surgeon. Your family doctor may refer you to the surgeon's office for an appointment, where you will have an opportunity to meet face to face. Or if the situation is urgent, the doctor may choose to admit you directly to the hospital, where you will meet your surgeon (one hopes) some time before the planned operation. In the latter situation, your doctor may not have selected a surgeon for you, considering your admission to be of prime urgency, preferring to defer the choice of surgeon until later.

Let us consider the first situation, where you are referred directly to the surgeon for a review of the need for an elective operation. During this interview, the verbal contract for surgery will be made.

It is worthwhile to consider what you might expect when meeting your surgeon and what you should look for.

Surgeons are different from other doctors, although they are physicians, too. And surgeons in one specialty are often of a different mold than surgeons in another.

WHAT TO LOOK FOR IN A SURGEON

In the public's mind surgeons have been portrayed as people having "the brain of an Apollo, the heart of a lion, a clear eye and a woman's touch." Others think of them as being egotists, megalomaniacs, cold and aloof, insensitive and unfeeling, whose prime concern is to wield the scalpel, with profit as their dominant consideration. Being a surgeon, I have heard most of these descriptions, but as generalizations, they are mostly untrue. Yes, most surgeons are confident. But I consider confidence to be one of the prime requisites of the profession. Without it, surgeons would never be able to handle the difficult or unexpected situations that they encounter. The self-confidence of a surgeon is seen in that jaunty stride along a hospital corridor, with white coat (and retinue) trailing behind. It is evident in manner, speech, in the surgeon's every action. It inspires confidence in those around him or her—assistants, nurses, and, most importantly, the patients. For who would want a surgeon who is indecisive, hesitant with uncertainty, lacking in self-confidence? Upon meeting one such, a patient would quite likely check out of the hospital on the spot. It is this quality in the surgeon that results in a patient, even after only the briefest of meetings, placing absolute trust in the human being who is about to perform a major operation on him or her. It is a remarkable thing indeed!

But self-confidence is often mistaken for arrogance or pomposity, brusqueness or lack of concern. When there is an excess of self-confidence in a surgeon, without personal insight into his capabilities or shortcomings, this can be a dangerous quality. Such a person may, with an aura of infallibility and omnipotence, embark on operations that carry unwarranted hazard to the patient, operations that are simply unnecessary.

Dr. Rudolph Matas, in an address entitled *The Soul of the Surgeon*, delivered over sixty years ago, described surgeons as follows:

> *They are the men who resort to all sorts of subterfuge to coax their patients to the operating table; they are the men who see in every cramp an appendix; in every belch a gallstone; in every heartburn, gastric or duodenal ulcer; in every uterus, a cancer or a fibroid; in the abdomen of every neurasthenic woman, a floating kidney or a prolapsed or displaced organ, that nothing short of an operation, a laparotomy, can cure or relieve—provided the patient can pay the necessary fee.*

Such a tarnished image of the surgeon still exists in many quarters, though I believe it is much less prevalent today than in years gone by. There are other characteristic traits of the surgeon that form a common personality pattern. For example, most surgeons are meticulous in their manner and dress, and this meticulousness often carries over into their home, making life miserable for spouse and children. Surgeons usually have the Type A personality, and in this instance A is not the equivalent of outstanding. The Type A person, according to Friedman and Rosenman, is a person who has an intense sense of time-urgency, always watching the clock, adhering to rigid schedules, an early riser, hustling about, on the go all the time.* He or she is impatient and doesn't like to be held up waiting for the anesthesiologist, the nurse, or the sutures. The surgeon

---

*Meyer Friedman and Ray H. Rosenman, *Type A Behavior and Your Heart* (New York: Alfred A. Knopf, Inc., 1974).

is always after the anesthesiologist "to get on with it" and is unable to relax. Basically, he or she is highly competitive in everything. Surgeons are forceful in their speech and often "rub people the wrong way." The behavior characteristics of the Type A personality are prominent among surgeons. Surgeons' fascination with numbers, statistics, the stock market is a common characteristic, as is their fascination with dollars. These are some of the recognizable traits of a surgeon, and I am sure my medical confreres could readily add others.

Affability and a pleasant, warm manner are very desirable qualities in a surgeon; unfortunately, they are not qualitites possessed by all. A surgeon's pleasant, relaxed manner in approaching a patient who is about to undergo a laparotomy for unexplained peritonitis is certainly of great benefit to the mental attitude of the patient. One of my colleagues, Dr. W. D. Smith of St. Michael's Hospital, possesses qualities of warmth and humor that are his trademark. His patients always feel better when he walks into the room. His laughter is infectious, and they share in his obvious enjoyment of life.

I consider the most important qualities of the good surgeon to be self-confidence, clinical judgment, diagnostic acumen, technical expertise, and compassion for fellow human beings. Of these, only confidence and compassion may be evident on the first interview. Unfortunately, many patients misconstrue intensity, dedication, and extreme concentration as an absence of compassion—aloofness. Don't expect your surgeon to gush all over you, to hold your hand, to be jocular or emotional. Most surgeons aren't built that way. But most are concerned, and most are compassionate.

What should you look for when meeting your surgeon? You should look for empathy and a willingness to communicate, to discuss your case. He or she should be willing to discuss your diagnosis, to determine whether more tests are required. If there is doubt about the diagnosis, the surgeon should be willing to consent to a referral to another consultant. If there is doubt about the need for surgery, he or she should agree to a second opinion from another surgeon. This is painful for most surgeons, I know, because it implies that a patient has less than complete confidence in their judgment. But most of us will concur in the matter, because to proceed without the patient's total acceptance can lead to difficulties later, in the event of complications.

Does your surgeon take the time to review your history? If he or she doesn't ask you questions about your previous health or previous operations and doesn't examine you even briefly, you just may have chosen the wrong person. If the surgeon doesn't examine your abdomen, or do a pelvic examination, or look at your X rays, he or she is relying strictly on hearsay information. How can there be certainty without checking? There can't! A failure to do any of these may be the basis for a complication occurring during the operation. (It is not unknown for a patient's only kidney to be removed, only to find that what was thought to be an ovarian cyst was, in fact, the patient's only kidney.)

It is not unreasonable to ask whether your surgeon has done the operation before (i.e., a liver resection, a pancreatic resection) when the hazard to you may be great—that is, when the operation carries a high mortality rate. Nor is it unreasonable to determine whether he or she will actually perform the operation personally. This is the only way that you can avoid having a "ghost surgeon" do your operation, unless of course the surgeon chooses to commit perjury.

WHAT TO DISCUSS WITH YOUR SURGEON

NECESSITY It is at this time that you might wish to consider alternative measures of treatment. Just how necessary is this operation? Is there an alternative to surgery—for example, medical treatment?

Let us consider three examples—duodenal ulcer, gallstone, and coronary-artery disease. At one time, the indications for operation for duodenal ulcer were (1) perforation, (2) obstruction, (3) hemorrhage, and (4) intractability or failure of medical treatment. The most common of the four was intractability, and operations for duodenal ulcer were among the most common procedures performed. Today, there is an alternative—a drug named cimetidine (Tagamet is its trade name)—that may heal your ulcer when other forms of medical treatment have failed. The frequency of ulcer operations has been on the decline, at least at our hospital, since cimetidine was discovered.

A solitary, noncalcified cholesterol gallstone may also, if small, respond to medical treatment. A drug called chenodeoxycholic acid may cause the stone to disappear in a fairly high percentage of cases, especially if it is a single, small stone. The stone may later reform, but at least there is an alternative to surgery.

Some forms of coronary-artery disease require surgical treatment—those in which the blockage is high, where the risk of a heart attack is great, and where symptoms are progressive and cannot be controlled by medication. There are other forms, however (stable angina, for example), in which medical treatment may be preferred, and a major operation (an A/C bypass) may be avoided. It is worth finding out if there are alternatives. I certainly tried medical treatment first.

MAGNITUDE The next most important thing that you should determine is the magnitude of the proposed operation. If you have a lump in your breast that you have been advised to have removed, you should determine at this point whether the simple removal of the lump will be performed or of the entire breast—a radical mastectomy. It is too late to wonder about it after the breast has been removed. Though I prefer to perform a modified radical mastectomy for breast cancer (and, it would seem, so do most surgeons in Canada and the United States), there are alternatives, with a small lump, especially in young women. But most of my patients know in advance that if cancer is found, the larger operation will be performed. Few have ever complained to me afterwards; most have reasoned that their life is more important than their breast.

If an operation for cancer of the bowel is under consideration, find out now if a colostomy will be necessary. There is no point in being bitter toward your surgeon later because he or she found it necessary to do one. You should have inquired to be better prepared. Many patients are disgruntled after surgery and claim "If I'd known I was going to be mutilated like this, I'd never have consented to the operation." These attitudes can be minimized by prior discussion.

Having been informed of the magnitude of the operation, you should determine other necessary things. The first is, what are the possible risks? What are the complications that can be expected in a certain percentage of cases? What is the possibility of not making it, of dying from the operation? And last, what will the cost be? Let us consider them in order.

RISKS First of all, the risks. It is necessary to define "risk." Broadly speaking, it is the probability of developing a complication; the complication may be nonfatal (morbidity) or fatal (mortality). Risk has been described as "slight," "special," or "serious," depending on the nature of the operation and the complication considered. For example, the risk of infection following an operation on the large bowel may be great, but the risk of death is slight. Also, "there may be slight risks of serious consequences and great risks of slight consequences."*

Let us consider the matter of the risk of wound infec-

---

*Gilbert Sharpe and Glenn Sawyer, *Doctors and the Law*. (Toronto: Butterworth, 1979).

tion following an abdominal operation, any operation within the abdominal cavity. The risk of wound infection in nonabdominal operations is in the neighborhood of 3 percent. In clean abdominal operations (i.e., gallbladder) it is nearly the same. In potentially contaminated operations (i.e., when the gallbladder is infected) the incidence of infection rises to nearly 10 percent. If a major resection of large intestine is performed, the incidence is higher—from 15 to 20 percent. If covering antibiotics are not used, the rate of infection may be still higher. Usually the risk is classified as "slight" but may be "serious," especially if the patient's resistance or general condition is poor. Among patients who are diabetic, obese, undernourished, or anemic, the risks of developing infection are greater, and the consequences may be serious. So the patient may contribute to or constitute the risk. If you have any doubts about the risks, you should ask about them. The surgeon should inform you of the risks (verbally), and for some high-risk procedures it would seem preferable to list them in writing on the chart or on the consent form. This is known as "informed consent," and it is part of the contractual agreement with your surgeon that you were informed of some of the possible dangers. As we shall see in a later chapter, failure to obtain informed consent has resulted in serious consequences, and large awards have been made to plaintiffs. It may be in the future that consent forms will require a listing of the complications of the operation and that these will be countersigned by the patient. A study of informed consent recently showed that when surgeon–patient interviews were recorded on tape, in approximately two out of three instances, the patient's memory for the details of the interview was deficient. It is only reasonable to expect that few of the details concerning postoperative complications will be remembered. It is only human nature to shut out unpleasant thoughts. But does this mean that the risks should be recorded and signed by the patient to truly represent consent? There is some disagreement on this point.

In the United States, there is no specific, consistent practice on informed consent. A representative of one hospital in northern New Jersey, however, put its policy this way: "Prudence and fear of litigation cause hospitals and physicians to give a great deal of attention to this [the matter of informed consent] and to have written documents describing the medical/surgical treatment and to obtain signatures from their patients."*

Sharpe and Sawyer, in *Doctors and the Law,* have this to say about informing a patient of risk†:

Thus, a decision to disclose these risks may be tempered by a number of factors. These include the gravity of the condition to be treated; the gravity of the known risks, both in terms of their likelihood and the severity of their realization; the intellectual and emotional capacity of the patient to accept the information without distortion of his ability to make a rational decision; the importance of the expected benefits of the treatment; and any other factors that reasonable physicians would judge to be relevant.†

However, the consent form will *not* be signed at this time, though it might seem preferable to do so. This is usually done the night before your operation, when you are in the hospital. So there is time to forget or misinterpret what the surgeon said; more of this later.

The second question we all ask ourselves, understandably, especially when confronted with a major question, is: "Will I come through the operation? Could I possibly die?" It is necessary to have some idea of the gravity of the risk, so that one may make necessary financial arrangements (or spiritual, for that matter) such as the preparation of a

---

*Office of the Administrator, Hackensack Hospital, Hackensack, New Jersey, September 1980.

† Sharpe and Sawyer, p. 38.

will or tidying up one's affairs. Though we may be assured by our surgeons that the mortality rate is less than 1 percent for the operation, many of us wonder whether we will be the one to fall into the mortality (obituary) column. As a surgeon, I am seldom asked this question; as a patient, I didn't ask since I knew the operative mortality rates. Like Dr. Nolen, I took the trouble to find out. But I try to tell my patients as gently as possible if there is grave risk or to assure them as firmly as possible when there is little or none.

I have used a number of terms so far in this chapter—*hearsay, informed consent, risk*—that imply a legal contract between you and your surgeon. Let there be no misunderstanding about it; although verbal to this point, that is certainly what it is—a contract. Therefore it is important that you understand a little more about risk. Every operation, whether major or minor, involves a degree of corresponding risk; the greater the magnitude of the procedure, the greater the risk of either mortality or complications. This is implied. But there are risks that you may reasonably anticipate and others that you cannot.

To illustrate, let us use the hysterectomy as an example. A wound infection will occur in something like 3 percent or less of all hysterectomies, no matter how careful the surgeon is in preparing his or her hands and in scrubbing the patient's skin. If you develop a wound infection, it is not necessarily the surgeon's fault. It is just part of the intrinsic risk. You were unlucky. Your surgeon is not automatically guilty of malpractice. You would have little chance of winning a legal action should you pursue one in such an instance. If a postoperative hernia developed as a result of the infection, that is also bad luck and part of the risk. Should your surgeon inadvertently divide a ureter while removing your uterus and complications develop, then it may be a matter of opinion as to whether that is part of the risk. Such a complication does occur, though rarely, even in the hands of the best surgeons. But if the surgeon was careful and deliberate and then encountered unexpected bleeding or inflammation, he or she would likely not be held at fault. If, on the other hand, there was no evidence of inflammation and nothing in the tissue specimen to suggest a problem (suppose it were normal?), and if the operative record indicated that no attempt was made to identify the ureter, that the operation was completed in twenty minutes (undue haste), and that the accident was not recognized, then you should not have to assume that the complication was unavoidable.

This is what a 1973 C. M. P. A. report has to say about urinary fistula:

> *The complication of urinary tract fistula at pelvic surgery is a mishap commonly reported to the Association ... most doctors when questioned will admit these difficulties can occur in the most competent hands. ... While the circumstances in any individual case will determine the defensibility of that particular action, doctors should realize that though damage to the bladder or ureter is an inherent risk of the procedure, if their work is poor, responsibility for harm done will be theirs. ... Further, when the indications for surgery are tenuous, any resulting complication becomes all the more difficult to explain and when the injury to important structures is something which should have been recognized by the surgeon at the time and was not, his position afterwards becomes less tenable. [p. 23].*

Furthermore, let us suppose that the infection in your wound was found to be the result of a retained surgical sponge. In this instance, the complication was not intrinsic to the procedure; rather, it was most likely the result of negligence. Usually, the principle of *res ipsa loquitor* prevails (the thing speaks for itself) in the case of retained foreign bodies, and usually no supporting evidence from expert witnesses is required to win an action should one be pursued. Let us consider the two categories in more detail.

UNPREVENTABLE OR UNAVOIDABLE COMPLICATIONS (THE INHERENT RISK)

In the foregoing example of the hysterectomy, I alluded to two types of complications—a wound infection and a divided ureter. There are many others that are part and parcel of the bargain. A few of the more common ones that may occur following any operation requiring an anesthetic are as follows:

1. *The incision—infection, hematoma, stitch abscess, wound separation, postoperative hernia.*
2. *The lungs—pneumonia, collapse, embolism.*
3. *The heart—irregularities of rhythm, myocardial infarction, heart failure.*
4. *The GI tract—distention, bowel obstruction, abscess, leakage of intestinal content, jaundice.*
5. *The kidneys and bladder—inability to void, reduced urine output, possible kidney failure.*
6. *The limbs—phlebitis, attack of arthritis or gout.*

It is apparent from perusal of this abbreviated list that it is as much the patient who is the risk as the operation. Though we do our utmost to prevent these complications and to reduce their frequency wherever possible, they cannot be entirely eliminated from the practice of surgery. They constitute inherent risk.

As has been pointed out, the risk of any of these complications increases in the elderly or the malnourished—undernourished or obese—and for diabetics or patients with skin infections, boils, or acne. For patients with preexistent lung disease, pneumonia is many times more frequent. Among patients with preexisting heart disease, high blood pressure, or heart irregularities, heart failure and heart attacks occur much more frequently than in patients with normal hearts; and the same holds true for phlebitis and embolism. Also, someone who has had previous bowel surgery or disease is more likely to develop bowel obstruction (from adhesions) or an abscess or leakage. One with previous kidney disease is more likely to develop temporary kidney failure—and so on.

At this juncture it might be best to consider what you as a prospective patient can do to minimize the risks that are inherent in your operation. Though none of these complications can ever be absolutely and completely prevented, they may be reduced somewhat in frequency by preventive measures.

Heading the list would be a two-week period of total abstinence from, or a marked reduction in, cigarette smoking. Postoperative pneumonia and atelectasis, wound disruption and hernia are minimized by cessation of smoking. A smoker's cough is highly dangerous to a patient's incision.

Weight reduction may be considered second in importance to stopping smoking. Some surgeons will not operate on an obese patient unless there has been significant weight loss prior to surgery, because obesity increases the risk of lung complications and wound infection. Besides, operating on an obese patient can be difficult for any surgeon. Why not make it easier?

Any skin infection—boils or abscesses—should be cleared up prior to entering the hospital. In-hospital staph (staphylococcal) infections can be minimized through this measure. Some surgeons advise their patients to use surgical soaps (pHisoHex) on the area of the planned incision to reduce the risk of the patient's own bacteria infecting the wound.

PREVENTABLE COMPLICATIONS

In the second category of risk are the preventable complications, a compendium of errors that often fall within the realm of malpractice or negligence. First let us define the two terms so that we understand clearly what they mean. *Malpractice* may be broadly defined as an error of commission, the performance of a procedure that fails to measure up to accepted community standards. On the other hand, *negligence* is generally considered to be an act of omission, the failure to do something in the care of a patient that is a commonly practiced procedure. Today, however, most malpractice actions are framed in the category of negligence.

In the category of negligence are errors in diagnosis, delay in diagnosis, and errors in judgment concerning treatment. Errors due to malpractice may include the leaving of foreign bodies behind, improper choice of antibiotics, and unacceptable postoperative results. For example, it is not reasonable to expect that an infant would suffer loss of the penis from circumcision; that a woman would suffer loss of a leg following varicose vein ligation; that permanent mental deficiency would follow a brief general anesthetic for removal of toenails; or that the wrong eye would be removed. These are all extreme examples of malpractice (all of which have happened) that fall within the preventable category of complications.

Your surgeon should be willing to discuss some of the potential risks that are inherent in any operation (the largely unpreventable kind—infection and so on) and those that are especially related to the operation planned (diarrhea following vagotomy—division of the nerves to the stomach—for duodenal ulcer, for example). It is unlikely that all of the preventable kind will (or should) be mentioned, so don't expect it. Were we to draw our patients' attention to the most horrendous complications, who would ever consent to having an operation?

The final question you should ask is this: "What will the fee be?" In the United States, surgical and hospital fees are extremely high. They can wipe out a family's life savings, especially of those who do not have at least some medical insurance coverage. Private insurance plans, such as Blue Cross and Blue Shield, and government programs, such as Medicare (for older people on Social Security), pay a standardized amount for various surgical procedures and hospital services. If your hospital and/or surgeon charges a fee that is beyond that amount, you will be responsible for paying the difference.

Fees for the selfsame operation vary widely across the country and from one surgeon to another, sometimes as a function of his or her credentials. They can range, for example, from $450 or less to $900 or more for a cholecystectomy; from $500 and under to $1,000 or more for a total hysterectomy; from $250 and lesser amounts to $550 or more for an appendectomy.*

Recently, a close acquaintance of mine underwent varicose vein ligation of one leg. The operation (elective, cosmetic?) was performed by a plastic surgeon. The Canadian hospitalization plan allows $90 for this usually simple operation. My acquaintance was billed for $800! This figure may well have been agreed upon by my friend and her surgeon, but if it was not, then she came in for a surprise indeed. You have nothing to lose by asking; you have only your money to lose by not asking.

*Charlotte L. Rosenberg, "Why a New Malpractice Crisis Is Coming," *Medical Economics*, October 29, 1979, pp. 109–114.

Finally, there are certain danger signs that you should be alerted to when meeting your surgeon. Beware of unusual payment arrangements. A surgeon doing elective cosmetic surgery often requests payment in advance, and tonsillectomies are usually half paid for prior to the procedure. Otherwise, however, it is *not* customary for the surgeon to bill for services until after they have been completed. Beware if your surgeon discusses fees before reviewing your diagnosis and the need for surgery; beware if he or she seems to be in excessive haste to operate or seems to be pressuring you; beware if the individual refuses to agree to a second opinion or a consultation or refuses to discuss complications and brushes your questions aside with guarantees of 100 percent success or cure; and beware if he or she refuses to discuss your fee at all. If you do not, you may be paying for your surgeon's next trip to Rome or contributing to the down payment on a Florida condominium. Or your family may cash in on your life insurance policy. What you should look for is interest, concern, warmth, compassion, and a willingness to discuss your case.

On the other side of the coin, the surgeon may be wise to refuse to operate on you! If you are obese, or elderly, or suffer from preexisting heart or lung disease, the risks involved in performing a major operation on you might be excessive—an unanticipated complication, an unexpected mortality, or a possible lawsuit.

When you are having an operation, you must be aware of the risks—both the inherent and the preventable ones—and you should consider them carefully. After all, it's your life that hangs in the balance.

6 Entering the hospital: the preoperative period

You have made the decision to have an operation; you have selected your surgeon and hospital; presumably, you have met your surgeon and have given verbal consent to the procedure. You have considered the risks and the costs. Part of the contract, the verbal part, has been established. But you have not yet signed the consent form—the written contract. This comes a little later.

PREADMISSION

First you will have to wait for a bed. If your situation falls into the emergency or urgent category, it is unlikely that your waiting period will be long. Your operation will be given preference over elective and cosmetic procedures. If you are among the elective group, do not be surprised if you have to wait a month or more for admission. Cancer patients and trauma cases quite naturally take precedence over patients with varicose veins and gallstones. Besides, there has been a decrease in the number of beds in some hospitals without a corresponding decrease in the number of surgeons, so the waiting lists are getting longer. In England, waiting lists of a year or more are not unusual for elective procedures, so don't despair.

Your waiting period may be longer if you have chosen a private room. In some hospitals these are at a premium. Two-bed semiprivate rooms seem to be the norm, as they are more economical from the hospital's standpoint. Four-bed units can hardly be called semiprivate any longer. They offer only a minimum of privacy, and bathroom facilities must be shared. Strictly speaking, these are ward accommodations. Anything larger than this? Eight-bed units *are* wards!

During this period of waiting, your doctor or surgeon may choose to order more tests and X rays outside the hospital so that all of these are completed before your admission. This makes good sense since it cuts down hospital costs and may serve as a check for possible complications.

Once you have been notified of your date of admission, you can make definite arrangements about notifying your employer, providing supervision for your children, and so forth.

ADMISSION

If you have been a patient at the hospital before, you will have a chart number, and this will be registered. Your chart will be drawn immediately and sent to the ward. Upon arriving at the surgical floor, you will be directed to your room and likely advised to change from your street clothes into nightclothes. Shortly, your weight, blood pressure, pulse, and temperature will be taken by a nurse, nurse's aid, or student. These form baseline readings for future comparison. If you have a Medic Alert necklace or bracelet, this should be drawn to the attention of the nurse. It may indicate that you are diabetic, epileptic, allergic to penicillin or horse serum, taking anticoagulants—any number of things. For obvious reasons, do not conceal your bracelet. You will be questioned about allergies to drugs, and any allergy will be listed at the top of your medication sheet.

You will be asked to provide a urine specimen and some blood. The latter will be taken by a hematology technician. It may involve only the prick of a finger (it hurts nevertheless) or the puncture of an arm vein with a needle and syringe. These provide baseline readings of your blood counts (hemoglobin and leucocytes), as well as a smear for microscopic examination.

A blood sample may be necessary for typing your blood and cross-matching with a donor of the same type if your surgeon orders it. Blood on standby is ordered for most major operations in the event that a transfusion becomes necessary. If all goes well, the blood may not be used and will be returned to the blood bank.

Should there be a history of jaundice, kidney disease, diabetes, or the like, more complicated tests than these may be required. Though it is discouraging to see a member of the Dracula Corps enter your room every day, most tests are necessary for your protection. Your bone marrow manufactures enough blood each day to make up the loss, so don't think you will be exsanguinated by the withdrawals.

If you are having a major operation under general anesthetic, whether you have a history of heart or lung disease or not, an EKG and chest X ray may be ordered. At some time during your first twenty-four hours you will have another history taken and a physical examination. In most institutions this is required by law. There must be a complete history and physical recorded on your chart before you undergo major surgery. If it was done thoroughly before admission, it may not be necessary to repeat it provided it is recorded on the chart. In larger teaching hospitals this is often done by a clinical clerk, an intern, or a surgical resident. It is an inconvenience, but a necessary one.

If you have not met your surgeon prior to admission

to the hospital, you should reasonably expect to do so now. For common elective procedures, his or her visit and examination may be cursory. The same considerations should go through your mind as those mentioned in the previous chapter. Primarily you should discuss what the operation will be and what problems or complications you might expect. In most instances, you can be certain, your surgeon will be most reassuring.

At this time, the surgeon may choose to defer surgery until more tests have been done—a sigmoidoscopy (examination of the rectum and lower bowel); liver, brain, or bone scans to determine if there has been further progression of your disease. Even for a gallbladder operation, he or she may choose to order an intravenous dye test to determine whether any stones have passed from your gallbladder into the bile-ducts. It may be necessary to repeat a test already done—a gastric series or barium enema, an IVP—to learn if there has been any change from previous X rays. It is better for your surgeon to be prepared in advance for complications or difficulties than to discover them during the operation, totally unawares.

Sometimes the operation must be deferred to insure proper preparation of the part to be incised—laxatives, enemas, and antibiotics for a colon operation; chest physiotherapy, breathing and coughing exercises, or inhalants and decongestants before a chest operation. A good surgeon doesn't rush in without insuring optimum preparation on the patient.

THE WRITTEN CONSENT

If your surgery is planned for the day following admission—quite a common practice for elective operations—you will be expected to sign a consent form for your operation. In the United States, consent forms differ from state to state

SPECIAL CONSENT FOR OPERATION OR OTHER PROCEDURE

Date: _____ 19 ____

Time: _____ AM / PM

1. I, the undersigned, a patient in Englewood Hospital, hereby authorize Dr. _____ and/or such assistants or designees as may be selected by him, to perform the following procedure(s):

_____

_____

(list procedure(s))

on _____
   (name of patient)   or   myself)

2. It has been explained to me that during the course of the operation, unforeseen conditions may be revealed that necessitate an extension of the original procedure(s) or different procedure(s) than those set forth in Paragraph 1. I therefore authorize and request that the above named surgeon, his assistants or designees perform such surgical procedure(s) as are necessary and desirable in the exercise of professional judgment. The authority granted under this Paragraph 2 shall extend to treating all conditions that require treatment and are not known to Dr. _____ at the time the operation was commenced.

3. I consent, authorize and request the administration and management of such anesthesia as is deemed suitable by the physician-anesthesiologist.

4. I acknowledge that no guarantees have been made to me as to the results of the operation or procedure(s).

5. _____   _____
   (Witness)   Signature of Patient

                                       _____
                                       Signature of Spouse

(If patient is unable to sign or is a minor, complete Section 6)

6. Patient (is a minor _____ years of age) is unable to sign because
_____

_____   _____
   Witness   Signature of relative or
                                       legal guardian

and from hospital to hospital. They include the name of the hospital, the patient's name, the type of operation proposed (cholecystectomy or hysterectomy, for example), the date the consent form was prepared, the name of the surgeon, and a place for the patient's signature (and that of a witness). There is commonly a section included that states two additional things: (1) that you consent to your surgeon doing whatever may be necessary should an unexpected situation arise, and (2) that you consent to whomever your surgeon designates to participate in or to perform your operation. Let us consider each clause separately.

In the first instance, a surgeon who finds that your appendix is diseased may decide to remove it in addition to the gallbladder or uterus; one who finds a tumor of the small bowel that can be resected without danger may choose to do so as well. You wouldn't want to find out later that you had to have a second operation for a condition that could easily have been dealt with during the first one. The consent form cannot cover every possible eventuality. It is designed to give your surgeon some leeway.

In the second instance, the clause is inserted in most teaching hospitals so that if a surgeon chooses, he or she may elect to have an assistant or resident perform a part of the procedure or the whole thing. This often consists of the assistant making the incision and closing it, but it may involve more. It presumes, but does not specifically state, that your surgeon will assist or supervise whomever is chosen to do the operation. As stated earlier, there is no other way for the surgeons of the future to learn surgery except by being taught. Even in such prestigious institutions as the Mayo Clinic, in this era of "team surgery," residents assist and often perform operations while being assisted. It is important that you know this. Difficulties may arise, not when your surgeon assists another, but when he or she leaves the operating theater altogether and is unavailable for consultation if something should go wrong. Unfortunately, you have little protection if your surgeon is not an individual of conscience. Leaving an inexpert, untrained surgeon entirely to his or her own devices to perform a difficult operation on any patient is unconscionable.

I was once involved in a serious matter when I was a young attending surgeon. I left two residents (one fully trained with his F. R. C. S.—Fellowship of the Royal College of Surgeons, the other eligible to write that year) to perform a relatively minor (there's that word again) operation, a colostomy, on an indigent patient with a nonresectable cancer of the bowel. I advised my residents to perform a simple loop colostomy to defunction the colon above the area of obstruction from the tumor, since the tumor itself was too extensive to be resected. At the operation they decided that instead of a loop colostomy, they would fashion an "end" colostomy, which necessitated dividing the bowel, oversewing the lower end, and bringing the upper end out through an opening in the abdominal wall. For one reason or another, either because of excessive length or tortuosity of the bowel, the bowel became twisted, and the residents inadvertently oversewed the wrong end; instead of bringing the upper end out through the skin, they mistakenly oversewed it and brought out the lower end. Of course, the patient became immediately obstructed, the bowel eventually perforated, and the patient died.

An inquest was ordered after an autopsy showed the true state of affairs. In my opinion, it was a definite case of malpractice in which the principle of *res ipsa loquitor* (the thing speaks for itself) could have been applied. The nature of the error was apparent to everyone in court, but why the error occurred was unclear, even though the details were completely aired. Because of superficial cross-examination of witnesses by the crown attorney and confusing medical testimony given by a surgeon acting as a "friend of the court," the jury failed to appreciate the fundamental error that was made and returned a verdict that no fault

> **INFORMED CONSENT**
>
> WE ARE REQUIRED BY LAW to inform you of all the possible after-effects and consequences of general anesthesia. They are listed below. This list can be discussed in more detail if you wish.
>
> nausea/vomiting
> sleepiness
> numbness/paralysis
> paresthesia
> brain damage
> coma/shock
> hives/rash
> death
> inflamed veins/arteries
> infection
> loss of fingers/arms
> loss of legs/toes
>
> heart failure/cardiac arrest
> liver damage
> pneumonia
> hiccoughs
> nose bleed
> pharyngitis
> tracheitis/sore throat
> kidney damage
> hallucinations/dizziness
> laryngeal edema
> circulatory collapse
> eye irritation
> swelling
>
> Signed _____
>
> Relation to patient _____
>
> I have read this list and understand it. I give permission to Dr. _____ to administer general anesthesia and to do the treatment required.
>
> Date _____
>
> Signed _____
>
> Relation to patient _____

could be found. I was fortunate indeed that a legal suit of the greatest magnitude had been avoided for what I considered to be flagrant malpractice.

Though a legal action was not pursued, both the residents and I, and probably the hospital, were all liable. It was a bitter lesson; it took a tragedy to impress on me the need for my physical presence as assistant during an operation (even a minor one) done by a resident.

Most consent forms do not list the potential complications that may occur as a result of the proposed operation, though some lawyers advise that they should. In some states, (California, for example) the complications are listed in detail. Some consent forms in the United States are merely ridiculous. They outline every known complication that can occur in the entire realm of surgery or anesthesia. This is "informed consent" carried to the extreme. No reasonable person could ever assimilate all of this detail. A patient signing it would have to be deeply under the influence of preoperative medication to do so. And, of course, any consent form signed while under preoperative medication—for example, immediately prior to surgery—would in all likelihood be considered invalid when contested in a court of law.

To be properly informed, though, it would seem that a patient should be informed in writing, since memory is deficient. This is what the authors of *Doctors and the Law* have to say about informed consent.

> *The responsibility for obtaining an informed consent should never be delegated. He (the surgeon) must be certain that his patient understands his condition, the nature of the proposed treatment, alternative treatments available, the risks and chances for success of the proposed and alternative treatments, as well as the recommendations of the attending physician. Where possible, the physician should obtain consent before the patient enters the hospital.**

It would seem apparent that there can be little alternative but to put much of this in writing.

---

*Gilbert Sharpe and Glenn Sawyer, *Doctors and the Law* (Toronto: Butterworth, 1979), p. 38.

In Canada as well as the United States, regulations regarding informed consent are not set forth in law. A bill introduced into the Ontario legislature in 1977, entitled *The Patients' Rights Act,* proposed that

> *no written consent by a patient to a surgical operation, diagnostic procedure or other form of medical treatment would be binding "as an informed consent" unless prior to signing, the person giving it had been provided with an information form signed by a physician setting out the nature of the patient's problem, the advisability of treatment, the objectives sought to be achieved by the treatment, and any alternative treatment suggested to the patient and the risks inherent in such treatment.**

Not surprisingly, lawyers for the Canadian Medical Protective Association (C. M. P. A.) are opposed to enlarging and defining the concept of informed consent. General Counsel for C. M. P. A. Charles F. Scott, Q. C., argues: "The important question to be answered is, does it advance the case of the patient?" His answer is an unqualified no. He further states that it would "crib and confine the doctor in the exercise of his duty so as to make it impossible for him to exercise *freely* and in his patient's *best interests* the skill with which his training and experience has fitted him [italics, mine]."* He quotes from an earlier judgment that the duty of the surgeon "does not extend to warning the patient of the dangers incident to, or possible in, any operation, nor to details calculated to frighten or distress the patient."

It would seem that the duty of the surgeon toward the patient lies somewhere between one extreme—of passing over the risks lightly or offhandedly—and the other—of detailing percentages for every possible eventuality.

*C. M. P. A. Report, 1977, p. 35.

In review, the elements of informed consent should include some if not all of the following.

1. Diagnosis and nature of the illness.
2. Proposed operation, surgical techniques to be employed, and prosthetic devices to be used (if applicable).
3. Risk of death resulting from the operative procedure.
4. Potential complications of operation and prosthetic devices.
5. Benefits of the proposed operative procedure.
6. Alternative methods of management and their chances for failure or success.
7. Acknowledgment by the patient of his or her understanding of all explanations and answering of questions.*

One's signature on the consent form completes the written contract, which may require the signature(s) of one or two witnesses as well.

It is surprising indeed how few surgeons ever examine the consent form and personally attest to its accuracy. Usually we rely on the nurses to prepare the consent form, present it to the patient, and witness it. The nurses in the OR are the ones who usually check it on the morning of surgery. But in the delegation of this authority and responsibility, the surgeon assumes full liability if it is inaccurately prepared and if legal action later results because of failure to provide informed consent. The nurse is seldom held responsible; the surgeon invariably is. In this matter, we as surgeons have collectively been remiss. I know that at times I have been.

*Bulletin of the American College of Surgeons, May 1977, p. 8.

MEETING YOUR ANESTHESIOLOGIST

Only slightly less important than the surgeon in determining the outcome of your operation is the anesthesiologist. More and more legal actions are being pursued against anesthesiologists than ever before. The mishaps that occur under anesthesia from faulty equipment, improper intubation, imperfect ventilation or oxygenation of the patient, and inattention often result in tragic consequences—cardiac arrest and brain damage. The rewards to patients from judges and juries in these cases are exceedingly (though not unfairly) high because the consequences of error are so disastrous. Malpractice insurance premiums for anesthesiologists are exceptionally high as a result.

At one time the surgeon was considered to be the captain of the ship in the operating room, but not any longer. He or she is more often required to defer to the anesthesiologist. Though the surgeon still may be considered the "star" of the production, the anesthesiologist is now the "director." Few surgeons would persist in a course of action against the anesthesiologist's advice. This change in attitude has been a long time coming. Some surgeons are still reluctant to defer to the anesthesiologist's opinion, often to their patients' detriment. Consider the following example.

Recently, as a surgical witness, I attended an inquest in a small community where a young man had died shortly after an operation. The surgeon charged the anesthesiologist with delaying the operation unnecessarily and blamed him for the patient's death. The anesthesiologist had steadfastly and properly refused to begin until he had given the patient preoperative fluids and supportive therapy, whereupon the surgeon called in another anesthesiologist. After an unsuccessful and questionable operation, the surgeon wrote on the chart that a contribution to the patient's death was a delay in administering the anesthetic. In truth, the patient was quite beyond surgical help, as he had extensive gangrene of the bowel and was moribund and in irreversible shock. The surgeon and the anesthesiologist, each thinking that he was in charge, blamed the other. My only comment at the inquest was that the most important person in the operating room was not the surgeon, not the anesthesiologist, not the scrub nurse, but the patient.

This is what Sharpe and Sawyer had to say on the subject: "Where differences of opinion arise during surgery, the surgeon risks liability if he fails to yield to the judgment of the anesthetist where the issue lies within the latter's area of responsibility."

In some hospitals, anesthetics are administered by specially trained nurse-anesthetists. Unfortunately, many anesthetics are still given by general practitioners who may have little training in the specialty and who may feel uncomfortable giving them. Years ago, I performed an appendectomy on a little girl in a small hospital in the country. The anesthetic was administered by a GP who gave the occasional anesthetic when "no one else was around." The operation, because of poor relaxation, was unnecessarily difficult and hazardous to my patient.

Unfortunately, you may not get to meet your anesthesiologist before your operation. Seldom does a patient (unless the patient is a doctor and requests a good one) have a choice in the matter. Yet it can be extremely vital to your welfare. At our hospital, an anesthesiologist sees all patients the day before major surgery. He or she reviews the past record of anesthetics and operations and goes over one's past history of heart or lung disease, looking for potential areas of difficulty. The anesthesiologist also conducts a cardiorespiratory examination and may check on whether a chest X ray or EKG has been done. After such a review, it may be decided that a general anesthetic poses an additional hazard, and he or she may elect to give a spinal or local anesthetic instead, usually discussing this with you beforehand. If the anesthesiologist is not happy that everything checks out satisfactorily, he or she may order more tests (for high blood pressure, for example) or advise that the operation be deferred.

In some hospitals a separate consent form relating to the type of anesthetic to be used, the name of the anesthesiologist administering the anesthetic, and possible complications of the anesthetic may be offered for the patient's signature (as shown in the informed consent form).

If everything is to the anesthesiologist's satisfaction and your operation is to proceed as scheduled, you can expect a few more routine procedures on the eve of surgery. These often include a shave preparation of the operative area (excessive hair simply gets in the way), possibly an enema, perhaps a pHisoHex bath, and, last, a sleeping pill. Both your surgeon and anesthesiologist want you to have a comfortable night's rest, and so do you. After all, the day of your operation is important, and you want to be in the best possible physical and mental state.

7 The operation

The morning of surgery is charged with expectancy and uncertainty, whatever the magnitude of one's operation. Second thoughts go through everyone's mind: "Am I doing the right thing? Can I back out at the eleventh hour?" This is normal. I am surprised that more patients do not change their minds at the last moment, but few ever do. The expectancy is heightened by delay—if your operation is scheduled for ten o'clock and you are not called to the operating room until eleven. It is unfortunate that every operation cannot begin promptly at 8 AM, the ideal time from everyone's standpoint—that of the patient, the surgeon and the OR nurses. But this cannot be; someone has to wait. This is a good time to get out a book and read.

PRELIMINARIES

Regrettably, during this seemingly interminable waiting period, patients cannot soothe their nerves with a glass of milk or juice. For obvious reasons, breakfast and all fluids will be positively prohibited on the morning of surgery. It is imperative that a patient's stomach be completely empty during the operation. Under anesthetic, during induction, or after awakening, a patient may gag or vomit; on a full stomach, the result can be disastrous—an aspiration pneumonia, for example. Unless the operation is very minor and is being done under local anesthetic, you will not be permitted to have breakfast or fluid of any kind.

When you finally get the call to the operating room, you will likely receive your first injection. This may be a tranquilizer such as Valium or Demerol, which will make you feel very drowsy, possibly euphoric. Combined with one of these will be a drug (Atropine, in many instances) that will make your mouth dry and increase your craving for a drink of water. These medications are necessary to permit a smooth induction under anesthesia and to reduce the risk of your heart acting up. You also may receive an antibiotic injection for prophylactic purposes, especially if your surgeon is concerned about the possibility of your developing an infection.

You will be met on the operating floor by the supervisor or the head nurse in the OR where your operation is to be done. He or she will check your wristband to be certain that you are the right patient. The nurse will check to see that your consent form is in order and properly signed and will make sure that your dentures (if you wear them) and rings have been removed. He or she will reconfirm the nature of your operation, the part to be operated on, and the side (i.e., right or left leg, lung, or kidney) and will ask you if you have had anything to drink or eat that morning. These checks are all necessary for your protection.

When you are finally moved into the operating room, you will be met by the circulating nurse, who may double-check all the foregoing details. You will then be assisted onto the OR table by an orderly and nurse. This is the most lonely period of all, because you have no one to draw upon for emotional support. Besides, the atmosphere *is* slightly terrifying—a cold, sterile room; everyone wearing caps and masks; bright overhead lights, complicated equipment, and machines all about.

ANESTHESIA

At this time your anesthesiologist or the assistant will appear. Your surgeon may stop in briefly and say hello, but not always. I invariably did so for several reasons: to reassure the patient that I was present, to identify my patient, and to confirm the part or side to be operated on. A little extra reassurance at this time is most appreciated.

The anesthesiologist will first start an intravenous, most likely in your arm. This will serve a double purpose. It will be the route by which you will be put to sleep—induced—with Pentothal or some such drug; and it will be your supply line for fluids, blood, or medications during the operation if they are required. By this time you should be so well sedated and tranquilized that you will have little perception of the pain of the needle. Next the anesthesiologist may apply electrodes to your chest and arms to monitor your heart during the operation. He or she may ask you to breathe oxygen from a mask while the preparation continues.

Then the anesthesiologist is going to put you to sleep and will tell you just that. This takes no more than ten or twenty seconds. It is smooth and quite pleasant—even merciful, for the anxiety and apprehension are finally over. The time for your operation has arrived—almost.

Before the preparation of your skin with antiseptic, the anesthesiologist may insert a tube into your windpipe—endotracheal intubation—which is then connected to the anesthetic machine. This is often one of the trickiest parts of the operation—directing the tube between the vocal cords into the trachea. It is done in all major operations for your protection.

During the operation, the anesthesiologist must have control of your breathing, and this can only be done if a tube is placed in your windpipe. The gas machine (like a respirator) can take over your breathing at a determined rate, and there is less danger of spasm of your vocal cords or any other obstruction to your breathing. He or she can be sure of the exact proportions of anesthetic and oxygen being delivered to your lungs. Because of the presence of this tube in your throat, one of your most noticeable symptoms afterward may be a sore throat. Many of my patients complained of it, but after two long major operations, I did not experience any soreness at all.

A word about anesthetic agents: Most people dread the nauseating smell of ether and the unpleasant aftereffects of anesthetic gases. Today's anesthetic agents are a far cry from the likes of ether and chloroform of former years. Most of these—fluothane, triline, and nitrous oxide—are quite pleasant and usually have few aftereffects. Most hospitals have banned flammable and explosive gases, so the risk to the patient from the anesthetic gas itself is infinitesimally low—certainly the least hazardous element of the operation.

At this time or just before, to facilitate the intubation, the anesthesiologist may inject a muscle relaxant as well. Another benefit of the relaxant is that it enables the surgeon to operate without having to struggle against strong muscle contractions, especially those of the abdominal wall.

To doubly ensure an empty stomach, the anesthesiologist may choose to insert a plastic tube into your stomach through one nostril. With this, he or she can remove any residue that may have remained from the previous evening's meal. This tube may be removed at the conclusion of the operation, but for many procedures, especially those on the bowel, it is left in place.

After all of these manifestations, the area to be operated on is finally prepared with surgical soap and skin antiseptics, and then the area is draped. At last, the surgeon can begin.

THE REALITY OF SURGERY

Let us consider the ideal.

> *It begins with identification of the patient, verification of the operation and confirmation of the side (right or left) or part (hip, knee or ankle). The ritual of preparation of the surgeon's hands and the patient's skin (asepsis and antisepsis) must be meticulous for the patient's own protection. The antiseptic solution used is less important than thorough cleansing of hands and the operative site. Gowning, gloving and draping follow established and time-honoured techniques and are coincident with the induction of anesthesia.*
>
> *The skin incision is of sufficient length to provide ready access to the operative area without requiring excessive tugging and pulling by assistants for exposure (incisions heal from side to side, not from end to end). Hemostasis is precise using a maximum of digital pressure and a minimum of electro-cautery or ligature. Only when skin bleeding has been controlled does the surgeon proceed to dissection of the deeper layers.*
>
> *The requirements for safe surgical dissection are: good exposure, good lighting, good anesthesia and a dry bloodless field. Dissection may then continue along anatomical planes. It is performed principally with the*

scalpel, occasionally with dissecting scissors, rarely by gentle finger dissection but never by tearing or pulling tissues with forceps. All structures must be identified before division. In this way a ureter will seldom be inadvertently divided or a common bile duct accidentally cut. If a disease process so obscures the normal anatomy that structures cannot be identified, then the surgeon must weigh the risk of injury of the structure against the value of proceeding, being mindful of two precepts: do no harm and discretion is the better part of valour. Sacrifices of a healthy organ or structure may be inevitable if the surgeon is to proceed with the formidable task of resection of an advanced cancer of the colon. This is the essence of surgical judgment during operations.

Whatever the operation, gentleness of touch, no more than a caress, extreme caution and scrupulous care take precedence over all other considerations. More accidents are the result of overconfidence than technical ineptitude. Again, neither excessive speed nor extreme sluggishness is in the best interests of the patient.

The avoidance of surgical morbidity and mortality are the foremost objectives of the surgeon. A cool head, a steady hand, a calmness in the face of the unexpected are all required in full measure to insure a successful outcome. The expertise in the performance of the suturing is quite likely the least important factor in the insurance of a good result.

Before closing the surgeon must ask himself two questions: (1) Have I done everything possible to help my patient? (2) Have I left anything behind (sponge, forceps, needle) that will do harm?

During closure of the incision, the strength and type of suture are less important than accurate approximation of tissues, free of tension or strangulation. The surgical dressing should be comfortable, dry and act as a barrier to, rather than an agent of infection.

Given these, the surgeon's skill should provide him with a great measure of personal satisfaction and you, his patient, with a pleasant, successful outcome.*

WHEN THE IDEAL ISN'T REAL

This is the ideal that every surgeon strives for—a satisfactory outcome. But the ideal objective is not invariably achieved, even when all of these precautions have been taken. What are some of the things that go wrong, that get fouled up?

ANESTHETIC ERRORS Let us begin with the anesthetic errors: most of these are in the preventable category.

1. *Faulty anesthetic equipment—valves and such.*

2. *Failure to check the equipment thoroughly.*

3. *Improper intubation—prolonged attempts at insertion of the tube, or insertion of the tube into the esophagus instead of the windpipe.*

4. *Inadequate oxygenation—too high a ratio of anesthetic to oxygen.*

5. *Improper monitoring equipment.*

6. *Failure to monitor patient's vital signs properly.*

7. *Overdose of muscle relaxants or other drugs.*

8. *Overloading with IV fluids; air entrance into IV line.*

---

*John A. MacDonald, M.D., *The Art of Surgery* (Toronto: Mission Press, 1976), pp. 104–106.

9. *Undertransfusing; transfusion reactions.*

10. *Abandoning patient (visit to staff room).*

11. *Aspiration of vomitus on extubation.*

12. *Too light a level of anesthesia.*

An example of one such error from the C. M. P. A. report of 1978 follows.

A 29-year-old woman, a highly paid professional person, married and with two children, had a laparoscopic tubal interruption procedure done under general anesthesia on the fourth post-partum day. Pre-anesthetic assessment was carefully done, the patient was in good health and the anesthetic was administered by a competent specialist anesthetist who induced anesthesia with Pentothal, carried out tracheal intubation following an injection of muscle relaxant and established assisted ventilation with a mechanical respirator. The anesthetic was maintained with nitrous oxide and oxygen. A cardioscope although available was not used because of recent difficulty with the electrode connections. *When anesthesia had been established and after the surgeon had introduced carbon dioxide into the peritoneal cavity and was proceeding with the laparoscopic operation in the darkened operating room, the anesthetist left his patient unattended to check the vital signs of another patient anesthetized in the adjacent operating room for abdominal surgery. When he returned after an interval which was likely no more than four minutes, he found his patient pulseless; the anesthetic was stopped, cardiac massage was started and the patient was ventilated with pure oxygen. By the time the cardioscope was attached to the patient there was evidence of good cardiac contraction and the blood pressure had stabilized at about 120 mm. Hg. systolic.*

In the early post-operative period it soon became apparent that the patient had suffered serious brain damage during the cardiac arrest, the precise duration of which could never be accurately determined. Speculation about the cause of the mishap did not lead to any certain conclusions. There was the suggestion that gas embolism might have occurred. Consideration was also given to the more likely possibility that increased intraabdominal pressure during laparoscopy, pressure in excess of the acceptable 30 mm. Hg., had led to a severe decrease in cardiac output resulting in cardiac arrest. Whatever the cause of the mishap, when a legal action was brought and the conduct of the anesthetist was carefully reviewed by experts, it ultimately proved impossible to support the anesthetist's legal position in the matter and a very large settlement had to be made, recognizing that a young, healthy, and productive woman had been rendered totally incapacitated. Although there was some recovery of cerebral function, the patient was not able to return to her professional activities and will require constant care by her family and perhaps permanent institutional care.

It was the anesthetist's absence from the room at the critical time which forced settlement of this action. It is well recognized that dangerous hypoxia can occur insidiously and that this and other complications can be difficult to recognize, particularly in a darkened room, but surely this is only additional reason for greater vigilance. Had the anesthetist been present throughout, the outcome in this case might have been no different. Nevertheless experts consulted were forced to acknowledge that constant attention and early rec-

ognition of the complication might have avoided the disastrous result. Nowadays simultaneous administration of two anesthetics by an unassisted anesthetist is a practice which should be abandoned entirely. [Pp. 13–14]

Another tragic example from the C. M. P. A. report of 1974:

A 25-year-old father of two, in good health, was admitted for surgery of a deviated nasal septum. Anesthesia was induced by nitrous oxide, oxygen and Penthrane, and after 100 mg. of Anectine produced relaxation, a No. 10 endotracheal tube was inserted without difficulty and was fixed to the patient's face with a piece of tape. A short time later the position of the tube was changed on the request of the surgeon. At about this time the anesthetist encountered some difficulty ventilating the patient. The endotracheal tube was found kinked and partially collapsed and it was manipulated from beneath the drapes; the drapes were not removed. The difficulty lessened but did not disappear. The operation proceeded, the patient requiring more relaxant to facilitate the release of bronchospasm. When the operation ended, twenty minutes after induction, a large amount of pink, frothy, bronchial secretion was aspirated, and about the time when the drapes were removed the patient suffered what appears to have been a momentary cardiac arrest which responded to external cardiac massage. A second arrest occurred in the recovery room and was promptly recognized and treated because the patient was then under close observation with a cardiac monitor. The patient survived but not without a major neurological disability which included almost total blindness, dysarthria, and a cerebellar syndrome involving all four extremities. When a legal ac-

tion was brought, and as the details of the anesthetic were reviewed, it became apparent the patient had been subjected to a significant period of hypoxia probably caused by obstruction of the airway by a persistently kinked endotracheal tube and which went unrecognized throughout the operative procedure. Damaging hypoxia leading to severe disability or death can go undetected beneath the drapes if the anesthetist is not alert. In this case, the anesthetist had been less vigilant than the circumstances demanded and a settlement had to be made. [p. 12]

Unfortunately, the consequences of anesthetic errors are often tragic—shock, heart failure, cardiac arrest—and because they often result from human errors, which are difficult to defend in court, judgments have increasingly been handed down against anesthesiologists for staggering sums of money.

SURGICAL ERRORS Since the variety and number of operations performed are in the thousands, to list all the mistakes that could occur would be nearly impossible, nor would it serve any purpose. Errors during surgery can be classified broadly into a number of general categories.

Errors in judgment: This may take the form of an error in identification—of the patient, part, or side to be operated on. Fortunately, these are uncommon. An error in diagnosis falls into this group—what is thought to be a benign lesion turns out to be malignant, or vice versa; what is thought to be a malignant tumor turns out to be benign, and an unnecessary extensive resection is undertaken. Judgment errors occur when the surgeon performs the wrong operation for that particular patient or disease. Judgment errors probably account for the majority of intraoperative mistakes.

Technical errors—errors of execution: Although malpractice lawyers tend to think that surgeons are ham-handed and bungle operations, the majority of malpractice suits do not result from technical errors. Cutting a vital structure such as a nerve, ureter, vessel, or bile-duct is more often the result of faulty judgment, inattention, or undue haste than the result of technical incompetence. There are relatively few malpractice suits that result from poor suturing, leakage of an anastomosis, failure of a graft, or breakdown of a wound for technical reasons.

A surgeon in Ontario performed three intestinal bypass operations for obesity on members of a single family. In all of them he hooked up the lower intestine incorrectly, and all three patients died. This was a technical error caused by imperfect knowledge of the anatomy or by inattention to the details of the simple hookup. The actual suturing was probably perfect.

Errors of omission: This covers a wide variety of things, including failure to do a complete exploratory to check for other diseases, failure to check for a sponge or instrument before closing. This comes under the category of negligence. States one writer on the subject: "The attention of lawyers and patients seems to many doctors to have shifted from acts of commission which hurt the patient, to acts of omission which are much harder to define and much more debatable in their effect."

This is not so, however, with a retained sponge or instrument. The act is clearly definable, and it is difficult to defend. Just how common is it? In Canada, for example, in 1967 there were reported to the Canadian Medical Protective Association only 130 retained foreign bodies among an estimated 1.5 million operations, so it is not all that common. Over 95 percent of these foreign bodies are sponges, forceps, drains, and needles, and half are left behind by general surgeons. As one might expect, the majority are left in the abdominal cavity following stomach and gallbladder operations.

In the case of lost sponges, the sponge count was reported as being correct 48 percent of the time! These sponges are usually discovered *after* the patient has left the hospital and within a year of discharge.

What is interesting about retained foreign bodies is that the patient or relatives were informed of the event in 84 percent of the instances. How many sued their surgeon? A hundred percent? Seventy-five per cent? It may come as a surprise that only 42 percent pursued legal action! Since 51 percent of sponges are left behind by gynecologists, it may be that a sound doctor–patient relationship has been the main reason that lawsuits were not pursued by more than half of their patients.

Standard practice on instrument and sponge count varies from hospital to hospital in the United States, but the general situation was recently described as follows: "Recommended practice by the Association of Operating Room Nurses is that instrument, sponge, and needle counts be done on all cases prior to the beginning of surgery and prior to closing in surgery. It is practiced in all hospitals throughout the United States but in different modifications."*

Should the patient be compensated for these errors? Most lawyers tend to think so. I once removed a hot water bottle from a patient's abdomen that had become inadvertently folded upon itself and was missed during closure by another surgeon who was on holiday when I came to treat his patient. An abscess and fistula were present, and it was necessary to resect a small portion of intestine. Neither the assistant (who was asked to wash the powder from his gloves) nor the scrub nurse (who was asked to get a special instrument from her back tray) was aware of what took place, for the foreign body was quickly flipped to the floor and later discarded. The patient was not told about the real

---

*Office of the Administrator, Hackensack Hospital, Hackensack, New Jersey, September 1980.

cause of his abscess. Did I do the right thing? Was the patient not entitled to recompense? What if he had died rather than recovered? What would I want done if I were the offending surgeon? What would I want done if I were the patient in whom the foreign body was left? These are many of the questions that I have asked myself over the years since this event occurred. Therefore, weighing all factors, I believe that I was justified in my action as far as protecting the surgeon was concerned, but not in my action as far as the patient was concerned.*

Was this patient entitled to recompense for his pain and suffering? I believe so. But I return to this subject later.

So the list of potential errors is infinite. It's surprising that they don't occur more often. But some errors never come to light. All surgeons (myself included) can recall errors—of judgment or commission—where there was potential liability. I take little satisfaction from the fact that I was never sued, because I realize that there were times when I might well have been. We all make mistakes, and it is often a matter of good luck more than anything else that we aren't sued at one time or another.

I asked a surgeon on our staff, one with over forty years of experience, if he had ever been sued. He said that he had not but that he had received one threat, which is quite different. The reasons for his remarkable record are that he has good surgical judgment and has the most pleasant bedside manner of any surgeon I have known. His patients idolize him and would likely not sue him even if he did commit an error.

From the foregoing account, one can appreciate the importance of choosing your surgeon and your hospital, one staffed with good anesthesiologists. It can be a matter of life and death—yours!

---

*MacDonald, *The Art of Surgery*.

8 The postoperative experience

Depending on the length of the operation and the hour at which it begins, a patient will usually regain consciousness on the afternoon or evening of the operation. My first realization that my operation was behind me occurred about 8 PM in the intensive care unit (ICU). This unit is an area of the hospital, usually close to the operating room, that specializes in care of the seriously ill, postoperative patients, serious trauma cases, and any patient who requires a respirator. Nearly all open-heart patients are sent directly to this unit from the OR, and they usually remain for four to seven days.

For major operative procedures that do not require the use of a respirator but do require special nursing supervision, patients may be sent to an acute care unit (ACU). Here, as in the ICU, the nurses are specially trained to handle major (surgical) postoperative problems—the management of chest drains, gastrointestinal suction apparatus, intravenous fluids, and so on.

There is little privacy in intensive and acute care units, and males and females are not segregated. The beds are lined up, six to eight to a unit; curtains from ceiling tracks provide the only privacy. However, when one is a patient in one of these units, one is usually too sick, too drugged, or both to notice or care. There is absolute equality of race, religion, and socioeconomic status in an ICU. During my stay, two other doctors and I were treated along with a truck driver, an insurance man, and a farmer.

For lesser procedures, one may regain consciousness in the recovery room, an area on the operating room floor where a patient is checked by a special team of nurses until he or she regains consciousness. From the recovery room, patients are usually transported back to their rooms on the surgical floor.

POSTOPERATIVE PROCEDURES

Of all three areas, the ICU is by far the most terrifying. I knew what it would be like in advance, because I had treated many of my own patients in the unit, and I was not looking forward to it at all. When I first awoke, the pain in my chest was indescribable, but I could not believe that it would be overshadowed by the pain in my leg, the area from which they took the vein grafts. I welcomed the pain, for it meant not only that I was alive but that my sensory system was normal—no idle wish. What I had dreaded even more than the pain was the endotracheal tube, the one in my windpipe that was hooked up to the respirator. We all have sensitive throats; that is why we gag when doctors put tongue depressors in our mouths. Mine has always been particularly sensitive. There was a constant urge to gag, one that even drugs could not suppress. Being conscious, unable to move or breathe on one's own, and being supported by a respirator hooked to a tube in one's throat is an unpleasant experience. What is most unpleasant of all is the stimulation of coughing by a plastic tube placed through the one in your windpipe and beyond. As soon as this touches the trachea, it feels like you have choked on a peanut—it results in instant, violent coughing. This is designed to loosen secretions in the respiratory passages to prevent pneumonia. These secretions are then aspirated by powerful suction through the plastic tube. The machines do your breathing for you, stimulate coughing, and provide a means of expectoration.

The forced coughing results in a strain to the wire sutures used in some kinds of chest surgery that approximate the divided halves of your sternum, with the result that you feel as though your chest is coming apart. Fortunately, there are powerful drugs—Valium, Demerol, and morphine—that quickly relieve pain and send you back into merciful oblivion. I have spoken to many patients who have been in the ICU, and most of them recall little or nothing of the experience at all. My recall for everything was most vivid, nearly total.

One should not be surprised after major or semimajor surgery to wake up with a drain in one's side. I used them often for abdominal operations, and they are routine in open-heart and chest operations to remove accumulations of blood, air, fluid—whatever. Sometimes they are connected to a water-seal drainage system and a pump, so that nothing can gain entrance to the chest (air) and cause lung collapse. These are usually removed when there is no further evidence of drainage and when X rays show the lung is fully expanded. They cause only minimal discomfort when they are removed. Drains serve as a safety valve for leakage of body fluids that could lead to later problems such as abscess or infection if allowed to remain in the chest or abdomen.

Nor should one be too surprised to find a catheter hooked up to one's bladder. In women with a short urethra, this causes little or no discomfort. In men, it is unpleasant, though not painful. It is necessary to monitor one's urinary output, which is a measure of kidney function. If this falls below a certain rate, there may be cause for concern. It is a divinely pleasant experience to have a catheter removed.

Nearly every patient in the ICU or ACU has an intravenous line, a plastic catheter placed in the neck (to the superior vena cava) or the arm for administration of vital fluids—salt, glucose, and blood. The IV line serves as a useful and quick route for the administration of narcotics for pain, for antibiotics, or for any other drug that can be given this way. Some patients have an intraarterial line, a catheter that has been placed in the artery of the leg for removal of blood samples (blood gases) to measure the degree of oxygenation of the blood and to determine how well they are getting rid of carbon dioxide. These blood gas tests can only be measured properly from arterial blood samples; hence the line in the vein cannot be used for them. They serve as a check on how effectively the respirator or your lungs are working, and they can quickly monitor serious trouble if it occurs.

It is apparent that nearly every orifice of your body is used for your protection. There may be a tube in one nostril (the gastric tube) placed into the stomach to prevent distention with air (either swallowed or from the respirator). Were this not present, an increase in gas cramps could occur later. It is used in nearly all operations on the esophagus, stomach, small or large bowel, pancreas, and liver. It causes irritation of both the nostril and the back of the throat, but at the very worst, it is merely unpleasant. It is a relief, though, when it is removed.

After the respirator has been disconnected and the endotracheal tube removed, oxygen may be administered through a nasal catheter or by means of a small mask that fits over the nose and mouth.

And last, there may be a thermometer in the rectum (they aren't the breakable type), connected to a thermistor so that immediate temperature readings can be taken.

What about your ears? These are assaulted by the constant beeping of cardiac monitors placed over the head of each patient's bed. The beeping sound is synchronous with the beat of the heart, so you hear 80 to 100 beeps per minute. plus the superimposed beeps of patients on either side of you. When someone else's beeping sounds became irregular, I thought my heart was acting up. It is a necessary cacophony of sound that is somewhat reminiscent of an ancient form of torture.

When everything goes well, the respirator and the tubes are removed in twenty-four hours, the drains in forty-eight hours, the catheter in seventy-two hours, and the arterial and IV lines about the same time. The gastric tube is not removed until flatus has been passed. At this stage, you are ready to leave the ICU to return to the surgical ward and your own room and bed. What a joy to see the light of day, to hear the beeping of automobile horns rather than heart monitors.

Surely all operations, you may insist, do not involve such a dreadful postoperative experience? Fortunaely, they don't. By comparison, the ACU is like a first-class hotel accommodation. There are no respirators and not as many monitors, so there is less beeping noise. There is usually more space, too. Here patients are usually conscious and aware of their surroundings. The nursing care in an ACU is no less efficient than that in the ICU. Usually, only the very best, most highly trained nurses work in the ICU and ACU.

If you are moved back to your own room from the OR on the day of surgery and have escaped the ACU, it usually means that everything went well, that there is little danger of immediate complications, that you are able to breathe and cough on your own. But coughing regularly will be expected of you. It is extremely painful, especially if you have an abdominal incision, and quite difficult to do with a tube in your nose and throat. It is at this time that you will understand the reasons for giving up smoking and losing weight prior to surgery. Smokers produce more mucus, and greater effort is required to cough it up. The obese and overweight simply do not have the muscle power to cough adequately and consequently are prone to develop pneumonia. At this time many smokers vow to forgo cigarettes forever.

There is another painful act that you will be required to perform—get out of bed. Depending again on the magnitude of the operation, this may be ordered for the evening of surgery or the morning afterward. It is necessary to prevent pneumonia in your chest and thrombosis in your leg veins. It seems unnecessarily cruel, especially when you hurt so much, but if your pain is severe, you'll get an injection of pain killer. This early movement will help you to void as well and allows for early bowel motility. Studies have repeatedly shown that early ambulation is the best safeguard against postoperative complications.

GETTING ANSWERS   Human curiosity being what it is, patients begin asking questions almost as soon as they are awake. Most want to know how the operation went; if a malignancy was found and, if so, if it was resected. Other questions asked are: When will the tube be removed from my throat? When can I eat or drink? When does my catheter come out? When do you take the needle out of my arm? When do you remove my drain? What about gas cramps? When do I have a bowel movement? When do my sutures come out? When do I get out of here?

We tend to give good news at once; it's good for the morale. We tend to withhold unpleasant news until the patient is feeling better. Suppose no cancer was found—then we tell the patient. If cancer was found and was resected, we usually say we found a tumor and we removed it; if it has spread, we withhold the news until later. A patient can only take so much in the first twenty-four hours. I try to restrain my residents from giving all the crushing details as soon as a patient wakes up. It is unfair, I know, since I was told my type of cancer within forty-eight hours of surgery. I nearly collapsed from the shock of the news.

I knew it was cancer, but to be told the type—one of the least favorable forms—seemed to be an unnecessary cruelty at this time. I wasn't ready for it. Discretion and compassion are both required of the surgeon when devastating news must be given to a patient.

With respect to the removal of the nasogastric tube, this will depend on your operation and your surgeon. Usually it will be removed when he or she hears bowel sounds with the stethoscope or when you have passed flatus. The tube is necessary as an outlet for swallowed air and helps to prevent distention and abdominal gas cramps. When the tube is removed, you will be allowed to take fluids for the first time—water, tea, or juices—and soon you can expect to have the intravenous removed as well. When you have taken clear fluids without ill effects, you may be given something light—Jell-O, custard, ice cream—leading up to a soft diet—mashed potatoes, minced vegetables, chopped meat. The final stage, a full diet, comes after you have managed these preliminary hurdles, so don't be too anxious to get into a juicy steak—your intestinal tract just won't be able to handle it.

Gas cramps usually mean that your intestines are lazy and can't work as easily as before. The cramps are uncomfortable, sometimes painful, but they can be minimized by early activity. Too much pain medication also tends to slow up the bowel, so giving it for gas cramps may be of dubious value. Similarly, drugs may delay the occasion of one's first bowel movement, and then laxatives or enemas may be required. So don't be impatient about this temporary change in your regular bowel habits. We have a saying among surgeons: "We never lose the battle of the bowels"; after all, Nature is on our side.

Catheters are removed when it is anticipated that a patient will be able to void independently. It is discomfiting to everyone—patient, nurse, and doctor—when we have to replace the bladder catheter because of a patient's inability to void. The abdominal muscles, weakened by surgery, are very important in the act of urination, and it takes time for them to regain their normal tone.

Drains, which I have already referred to, usually come out when it is evident they have served their purpose and all drainage from them has ceased. Some surgeons remove them gradually, shortening them an inch or two at a time, whereas others remove them completely. In some situations (i.e., mastectomy or skin graft) the drain may be left in for as long as eight to ten days to prevent the accumulation of fluids beneath skin flaps. The drains are then removed along with the sutures. In some gallbladder and kidney operations, drains (T tubes, catheters, and so on) may have been carefully placed in ducts during the operation (bileducts, bladder or kidney, pelvis, ureter) and are used for extra protection or for the purpose of taking X rays. If these show that everything is satisfactory, then they will be removed. In rare instances, patients may be sent home with tubes in place for specific purposes.

The timing of the suture removal varies. Today, we have many ingenious techniques available to minimize the discomfort of suture removal. In some situations we use an absorbable, intradermal suture that need not be removed at all; in other cases, it is a wire suture (favored by orthopedists) that can be pulled out easily—when a cast is removed, for example. For small incisions we frequently use sterile adhesive strips (Steri-Strips) that hold the skin edges together without any stitching at all. The era of metal clips and heavy stitches that cause pain when they are removed is passing into history. The stitches may be removed in the hospital, the clinic, or the surgeon's office, depending on the length of your hospital stay. Plastic surgeons prefer to remove sutures about the face early to minimize scarring; general surgeons, in a week to ten days; and orthopedists may leave them in until a cast is changed.

From the foregoing it will be apparent that a lot of monitoring is done for a patient's protection. It is the duty of the nurse to record regularly a patient's vital signs—

temperature, heart rate, blood pressure, and respirations—as well as the intake and output of fluids—intravenous fluids, urine output, and the amount of drainage from the tubes and drains. These records are kept on the patient's chart. Nurses' notes serve as a permanent record of one's progress, level of consciousness, amount of pain, and any untoward reactions. When something goes amiss, it is his or her duty to report the incident to the attending doctor. Nurses' notes are extremely important, as has been shown repeatedly in the courts. The courts have often preferred them to a surgeon's memory of an event when making decisions in regard to negligence.

Postoperative visits from one's surgeon vary from case to case and from surgeon to surgeon. For minor and semimajor procedures, the surgeon may visit the patient infrequently or not at all. For major procedures, daily visits are the rule until the patient has progressed out of the danger period. In teaching hospitals, residents usually visit every patient once or twice daily. One shouldn't be surprised by the absence of one's surgeon in the postoperative period. If complications do arise and the surgeon fails to check them out, he or she may be setting the stage for a negligence action. Most surgeons, though, rarely abandon their patients in the postoperative period. But don't expect to see yours every day. I didn't see my surgeon more than once or twice, but I knew that I wouldn't, either, nor was I concerned about it.

COMMON POSTOPERATIVE REACTIONS

One can expect certain reactions to surgery that do not qualify as complications but that may cause concern. They are part of the body's metabolic response to surgery. Any patient who has been in the hospital for a week or more following an operation can expect some, though not all, of these body changes.

The first is loss of weight. It follows that if a patient has been off food for three or four days, all of that individual's energy needs will *not* be supplied by intravenous feedings alone. The body draws on fat and protein stores for caloric energy; hence there is a slight loss of weight, which is usually quickly regained. I lost fifteen pounds in ten days following open-heart surgery, but only a pound or two after my lung operation. For minor operations there may be no weight loss at all. Part of the reason for the weight loss may be a temporary loss of appetite. This may persist for four to six weeks after discharge from the hospital, but it is seldom permanent. There is no better solution for it than a return to one's normal diet at home.

Sleeplessness is a common complaint of many patients and may necessitate the use of mild hypnotics or tranquilizers. It is natural to wonder, when lying awake during the night, if anything might be amiss. A good night's sleep alleviates anxiety during the day.

A brief period of depression is not at all unusual. I tell my patients that it is a normal reaction. Seldom is psychiatric consultation necessary. Assurance, understanding, and a mild tranquilizer or mood elevator are all that's required for relief.

What engenders most concern is the disturbance in bowel functions that may persist after leaving the hospital. If one is taking analgesics (many contain codeine) for pain, one can expect a definite slowing of bowel function. A gentle laxative or stool softener may be all that is necessary to overcome intestinal sluggishness. Once analgesics are stopped, bowel function should return to normal.

GOING HOME

The final question is, when do I leave? One's departure from the hospital varies, again according to the operation and how well you have done. We decide on the basis of your temperature (normal); whether you are free of pain, up and about, eating a normal diet, voiding on your own, and having normal bowel movements. Otherwise, your stay may be prolonged. If you have developed a complication—whether unavoidable or preventable—your stay may also be prolonged.

A word of caution: Don't be too anxious to return to work after your operation. Better to allow an extra two weeks more than you anticipated, especially for a major operation. It may be six weeks to three months before you will be able to return to physical work; four weeks for a sedentary job. This will vary, of course, depending on the nature of your job and the magnitude of the operation. For a spinal fusion it may be six months to a year before a laborer can return to heavy construction work. Someone with a desk job may be back in the office in two months.

It may be wise to plan a brief holiday after surgery to recuperate. It is good psychotherapy, too. Many of my patients head for warmer climates in the winter after having gallbladder surgery. This may be the time to cash in on some of your accumulated sick leave.

COMPLICATIONS   From this brief review of a normal postoperative recovery, it can easily be appreciated that there are many areas in which complications can occur, complications that are inherent in any operation (see Chapter 5). One can understand now why postoperative pneumonia is so common and why coughing is so important to prevent it; one can see the need for early ambulation to prevent the dreaded complication of pulmonary embolism. A review of the variety of complications listed in Chapter 5 may be useful here. It is worth reemphasizing that you, the patient, may *be* the risk; your complication may be the result of poor general condition. However, if this were invariably the case, we would have no malpractice problems. Unfortunately, we have the second category of complications to consider—the preventable ones.

Consider the following: A healthy woman, aged forty-seven, underwent a hysterectomy and ovariectomy—considered "routine." There were no operative difficulties. However, she did not do well after surgery. She was in constant pain and required Demerol up to the day of discharge; she vomited and became distended; she did not pass flatus and did not have a normal bowel movement; she spent restless, sleepless nights; her temperature was elevated. Though she was examined once by a resident and once by her gynecologist, no X rays were taken. She was discharged and continued to vomit at home. She was reassured by her surgeon over the telephone. A week later she was readmitted in great distress; peritonitis and gangrene were diagnosed along with complete bowel obstruction. An immediate operation was performed; all but four feet of her small bowel was gangrenous and had to be resected. In another twenty-four hours she might well have been dead. Recovery was prolonged because of a bowel fistula; a permanent short-bowel syndrome resulted that necessitated permanent vitamin B-12 injections and medication for diarrhea. The patient eventually recovered but with permanent disability. Her case is presently before the courts. The gynecologist will have great difficulty defending himself against a charge of negligence for inadequate and negligent postoperative management. His failure to recognize or treat an obvious bowel obstruction will be costly.

Any patient who has been through a major operation and then must endure a complication that could easily have been prevented naturally seeks redress.

9 From patient to litigant

An attitude prevails in our society today that every wrong must be righted; every slight, redressed. The adversary system flourishes on these premises. True, there should be an avenue for receiving legitimate and commensurate compensation, and no one would suggest that the system be eliminated. But the concepts of commensurate compensation as fostered by labor unions, human rights organizations, judges, and juries have taken firm hold in the public mind. People want something for nothing if they can get it; it's just human nature. We are increasingly becoming a more compensation-oriented society. The U. S. Ambassador to Britain, the Honorable Kingman Brewster, called today's welfare society "the entitlement state," meaning that its individual members feel entitled to secure for themselves as much as they can.* Malpractice suits are a reflection of this attitude; they are increasing in number every year in the United States and in Canada.

A special supplement to the *Bulletin of the American*

---

*A. C. S. Bulletin, November 1978, p. 11.

College of Surgeons entitled *A Status Report on Professional Liability,* states:

> *It is no exaggeration to label the situation a crisis. Granted the problem has been with us a long time, steadily growing worse, but recent events have escalated its seriousness in a dramatic way. Most urgent is the issue of insurance availability. It is one thing to pay high premiums, the term in these days of inflation is a relative one, and even when these are projected to absurd levels such as $50,000.00 or more per year, they are theoretically capable of being paid out of clinical earnings, if physicans and the bill-paying public can develop an extreme degree of financial tolerance, but when absolute unavailability of professional liability insurance threatens one or several states, with the imminent risk of shutting down the provision of service to patients, no one can characterize the term "crisis" as overdrawn.* [P. S-4]

There are a minimum of four participants in a medicolegal drama—patient, surgeon (or doctor), lawyer, and judge (or jury), and all four have contributed to the increase in litigation. The surgeon is not the only culprit. Let's examine each of them separately.

THE LITIGIOUS PATIENT

There are certain psychological characteristics common to litigants. Their personality patterns, though not uniform, are still commonly seen among the litigious minded. They show paranoid features and are often aggressive and hostile. Some may actually hate doctors, may feel that they have been "mutilated" (an expression often used) by their surgeon or that surgeons make too much money. They are not easily pleased, nor do they accept explanations readily. We have all seen them. They write threatening letters, and they cause concern to all doctors. We have to live with them. This is not to suggest that all patients who sue are paranoid or actually schizophrenic—by no means. The majority are not, but we must recognize those who are.

Not long ago I operated on a man for a recurrent hiatus hernia. He had been a patient in the hospital on many occasions and had received psychiatric treatment. Three or four different psychiatrists had labeled him a paranoid schizophrenic—hostile and subject to delusions of persecution. The operation was done for severe complications and was a complete success. His incision was closed with a suture that had incorporated in it a tiny ring that allowed the suture to be looped through the ring. The metal ring, as part of the suture, remained in the incision—but outside the chest cavity. It caused no harm. It was "discovered" by the patient when a chest X ray was taken months later by his family doctor. The doctor said to him: "You have a foreign body in your heart." The ring was superimposed over the outline of the heart on the X ray, creating the impression that it was actually in the heart.

One can imagine what thoughts this pronouncement evoked in the patient's mind—a retained foreign body, malpractice! It wasn't long before a writ was received from a lawyer, statements of claim were filed, and the issue was taken to an examination for discovery. The doctors, residents, OR nurses, radiologists, chiefs of staff, and the hospital were all named in the action. Although there was little likelihood of a successful outcome, the lawyer pursued this action in the face of abundant evidence that there was no foreign body in the heart or chest—that it was part of the suture. There was not a shred of evidence of malpractice or negligence.

On another occasion, an obviously mentally disturbed patient fractured his sternum (breastbone) in an accident.

The fracture healed, but it left a prominent bump on his breastbone. He asked me to repair it, as it was aesthetically unpleasant to him, though not painful. I refused because nothing was to be gained. He requested another consultation to which I willingly agreed. The second surgeon elected to placate the patient and straighten the bump. I warned him that if he did so, he could expect to be sued, no matter how good the surgical result. And he was sued, though not successfully.

These are extreme examples, to be sure, but cases like them do cause surgeons considerable consternation. We tend to blame the patient and the lawyer whenever we are faced with nuisance suits. It doesn't take many of these before the surgeon, too, becomes paranoid, since he or she rightfully feels persecuted.

Another area of potential difficulty is the unreasonable expectations that patients often have for surgery. When these are unfulfilled, there may be bitterness. If there has been unrelieved pain or unexpected pain, patients may harbor resentment, especially toward the nurses and doctors, if they think the health professionals weren't sympathetic or didn't care.

The patient may harbor unexpressed guilt feelings, especially in the area of cancer—guilt for not seeing a doctor sooner, guilt because of a delay in diagnosis. This guilt is often expressed as anger that is directed against the health care team. If there has been excessive pain and suffering in a terminal situation, members of the family may feel guilty and show hostility to the doctor or nurses.

The surgeon should be hesitant about operating electively on patients who have been injured in motor vehicle accidents and are in the process of seeking compensation for their injuries. Such patients may wish to extend the length of their disability as long as possible, and they may seek, as an ally in their attempts, a surgeon who is willing to operate on them for their complaint. A surgical operation may represent their proof of disability in court, even if the operation was a varicose vein ligation, a hemorrhoidectomy, or dilatation and curettage.

It is surprising how many patients will relate symptoms to an event such as an accident or a fall—whether it be hemorrhoids, a lump in the breast, or a back problem. If they feel they can be compensated for their pain and suffering and if they can find a lawyer who will take their case, they will instigate litigation. Two sisters, both in their fifties, successfully sued a driver who collided with their vehicle—one because her menstrual periods stopped, the other because her periods started again.

I recall seeing a patient with normal myelograms who, nevertheless, underwent laminectomy by an orthopedic surgeon for back pain and then refused to work because she was not 100 percent improved. This case took years for the courts to settle. A lawyer states: "The claimant's desire for reward frequently affects his trustworthiness and his subjective complaints. It is for this reason that the physician must be extremely thorough and objective."*

Poor communication between patient and doctor is a source of concern. Failure to understand the consent form or to receive informed consent is a common source of litigation. Consider the following illustrative cases.

In mid-1971, a 19-year-old married woman was referred to a surgeon because of lower abdominal pain of two weeks' duration; the patient had been married four years. She had wished for children but had not become pregnant even though no contraceptive measures had ever been used. The surgeon felt the cause of the trouble might be inflammatory pelvic disease, and after treatment with antibiotics had proved ineffective he decided

---

*Gravenor Colina Jr., "Medicine and the Law," *Canadian Doctor*, February, 1975.

exploratory surgery was necessary. He so advised the patient and, he said, informed her that if the site of the inflammatory disease were her tubes he might have to remove them. The patient seemed confused and was depressed after the explanation—so much so that one of the nurses suggested the doctor should interview the patient again. He did and he left satisfied the patient understood what had been told to her.

The nurse on the floor whose responsibility it was to have a consent for surgery signed readied the form for signature, went to have the patient sign it but deferred doing so because the patient had visitors. That nurse, then, went off duty. It was never possible, afterwards, to find any nurse who remembered having taken the form to the patient for signature; no nurse could be found who remembered witnessing the signature although at least two nurses were sure they saw the completed signed form on the chart. The nurse on the floor responsible for seeing that charts were complete before patients went to the operating room thought she remembered seeing the form; the operating room nurse responsible for reviewing the chart thought she saw the completed form. The doctor did not check; he assumed the form must have been completed and would be on the chart. The consent form was never found.

At operation both fallopian tubes were found inflamed, of tremendous size, "like big bags of pus" and both were removed. The morning after the surgery the patient asked what the doctor had done, and he told her. He told her as well that the severity of her disease probably would have prevented her ever becoming pregnant anyway and that if he had not removed the tubes, she probably would have required an operation later and probably fairly soon. A few days later the patient suggested that she had not understood, she never would have given permission and that, in fact, she never did give consent. She and her husband asked to see the consent form she allegedly had signed. It was then discovered no consent form could be found.

Claiming lack of consent, the patient brought legal action against the doctor. The claim came to trial some three years after treatment. The judge, summarizing the reasons for action, noted the clinical background, noted that a certain diagnosis could not be made without an examination under anesthesia, noted that "the evidence establishes, at the least, that she would be taken to the operating room———, the defendant would endeavour by examination to ascertain the nature of her problem. The plaintiff knew that if the problem involved her reproductive organs she might be rendered sterile. She was in a state of great anxiety because bearing children was a matter of utmost importance to her." The judge said, "The evidence clearly established that whether the fallopian tubes had been removed or not, they were in such a diseased condition that it is highly improbable that the plaintiff would ever have borne children—The plaintiff while admitting that she agreed to an internal examination under anesthetic, denies that she consented to surgery and particularly denies that she consented to the removal of her fallopian tubes—." There was, then, the doctor's second interview with the patient about which the judge said: "I can only assume that she wished to be assured that she would not become sterile or at least discuss the matter further before making a decision. The defendant saw her again but does not say she gave her consent for the removal of her fallopian tubes or the loss of childbearing capacity. He did not ask for her consent but merely told her he would endeavour to ascertain her problem and correct it." The judge went on: "The operation which was performed by the defendant was not an emergency operation and was not necessary to preserve the life of the patient. The defendant does not take the position that consent was unnecessary because of emergency circumstances."

The judge reviewed previous legal actions and decisions at some length and said: "It is contended that it is impractical and unfair and too high a standard of care to impose to say that a surgeon who finds infected organs as the defendant did here, must close the abdomen and seek fresh instructions. But that is not the standard debated here. The standard here is that in the absence of emergency the consent of the patient to an operation and to its consequences must be sought and obtained before the operation begins. An inadequate explanation of bare possibilities will not suffice. . . .

"I have found this a difficult decision to make and particularly so because I realize that (the surgeon) was, in his own mind, exercising judgment in the best interests of his patient. He assumed consent rather than obtaining it. He also assumed that the nursing staff had obtained it for him. Such assumptions are human errors which are understandable but which, unfortunately, do not justify the failure of duty which I have found present here."

The judge, in deciding on the matter of damages, made his decision on the basis that the patient had suffered shock and emotional upset, though "on the other side of the ledger she has been relieved of the risk of further infection and attendant damage and pain." The surgeon assumed consent in the case rather than actually obtaining it in writing, and his failure to have such consent resulted in an award to the patient.* [p. 104]

*T. L. Fisher, "Implied Consent Is Not Enough," *Canadian Medical Association Journal*, January 11, 1975.

From patient to litigant 123

The following represents a similar misunderstanding with regard to consent:

In 1964 a 42-year-old man reported to a general practitioner because of backache which had been present, with variable intensity, since a severe injury in 1961; in 1965 there was more complaint and radiography revealed an old fracture of the proximal phalanx of the large toe; for this the patient, later, was referred to an orthopedic surgeon who felt fusion of the toe was necessary. Nothing was done however until a year later when, as a result of more pain in the toe, the fusion was planned but deferred about three months at the patient's request. By the time the action came to trial some years later, memories differed of events and of their timing. The surgeon thought he remembered that during the three months' delay the patient's complaints about his back had taken precedence over those about his toe and thought he admitted the patient on the clear understanding that fusion of his vertebra was to be done. The patient, on the other hand, thought he clearly remembered having been admitted to have his toe fused. The doctor was insistent that he had stated clearly that the admission was to have surgery done on the back; the hospital records nevertheless talked of surgery for the toe. The doctor remembered talking to the patient the preoperative evening and getting his verbal consent; the patient had no memory of such an interview and steadfastly said he would not have consented to an operation on his back. The consent form was one of the . . . forms which ostensibly authorizes a surgeon"—or his assistants to perform such treatment as he in sole judgment and discretion shall think advisable." No mention was made of what treatment or surgery the surgeon in his sole discretion had advised or proposed doing. There was no evidence that the doctor either had the patient sign a consent form or checked to see if one was signed.

The judgment in this action hinged on the matter of credibility; repeatedly the judge seemed to prefer the testimony given by the patient. In the course of the judgment the judge made two things clear: "The plaintiff makes no suggestion that (the surgeon) . . . is anything but the reputable and well-skilled surgeon the evidence appears to indicate that he is. He does not attack his integrity. That he brought to the surgery he did perform the amount of knowledge and skill necessary for the task is not gainsaid . . . (the plaintiff) . . . did not appear to me to be vindictive, nor did he appear avaricious, nor ready to exploit the situation to his pecuniary advantage. . . . (The surgeon) . . . , as has been stated, appears to be a reputable skillful surgeon . . . the court has no reason to seriously question his integrity. I do, however, emphatically question his recollection in a number of instances with relation to the facts in the instant case. In some it is wholly defective. . . . In the light of all the circumstances disclosed by the evidence which I accept, I find that the plaintiff did not give his consent to the operation performed by the defendants. . . . I accept his evidence when he states that the spinal operation was not discussed with him prior to its performance."

The consent form did not specify the procedure to be undertaken but authorized the surgeon or his assistant "to perform such treatment that he in his sole judgment and discretion shall think advisable" and did not mention the operation the surgeon advised or proposed. The judge found the plaintiff had not given his consent to the spinal operation performed by the surgeon. The judge stated: "In the instant case I find that the onus of establishing a sufficient and effective consent rested upon the defendants and they have not met or discharged that onus. I am satisfied that there was, in fact, no consent given by the plaintiff for the surgery in question." He further ruled that the plaintiff was entitled to be compensated for damages.

Many doctors believe that it is a breakdown in human relations that is the primary cause of malpractice suits. Notwithstanding all the foregoing, there is always an incident or a complication that captures the patient's attention. It is difficult, even for doctors, lawyers, and judges, to distinguish between a complication that is unavoidable and one that is preventable. And so, too, for patients. They understand little about inherent risks or that they personally may be the risk. A patient has an operation, a simple one perhaps, then develops a complication and naturally assumes fault on the part of the surgeon.

A young man had a double hernia repair. The surgeon used silk sutures in the operation. The patient developed infection (staphylococcus) in both incisions that persisted for over a year. He went to a lawyer, and I was asked for an opinion. The young man suffered from severe acne of his face and back (due to the same staph). His wound infection was caused by his own bacterial organisms. It cleared quickly when the silk sutures were removed. The original surgeon could hardly be held responsible for the infection; the action was dropped.

Another hernia patient had wire sutures put in by a surgeon at a well-known hernia clinic: his work was impeccable. But after surgery, the patient developed pain during intercourse and was certain that it was caused by his sutures. The surgeon, on the other hand, was adamant that his sutures were not causing the pain and refused to remove them. The patient considered suing the surgeon, which I felt was inadvisable. His pain was relieved by removal of the wire sutures.

Some complications, though they may constitute inherent risk, are far more serious and tragic than these and naturally lead to wonder on the patient's part about seeking redress. One patient of mine developed postoperative jaundice from a transfusion reaction. He was very ill, and recovery was extremely slow. Another doctor suggested to him that there might be "an abscess in there, or an injury to his bile-duct." The germ of a malpractice suit was immediately implanted. Fortunately, despite repeated attempts by the patient's wife to instigate a lawsuit, no lawyer in Toronto could be found to take the case. This complication is another example of inherent risk, an unavoidable but infrequent reaction to blood transfusion.

Another tragic example was that of a young girl aged fifteen, a patient of mine, who died of liver failure after a "routine" appendectomy. A coroner's inquest was held to determine if the anesthetic agent used was responsible for her death. After a considerable body of expert opinion, it was determined that such was not the case—a disastrous consequence of "routine" surgery, but no liability on the part of anyone was involved.

A better understanding by patients and lawyers of what constitutes inherent risk and unforeseeable complications can lead to a reduction in nuisance suits.

Another common source of unfulfilled expectations is the matter of pain and/or deformity following the setting of fractures. Patients expect perfect results, and when there is less than perfect alignment, a deformity in the form of a bump or callous, they may seek legal opinion. Many inquiries are made in this area. Unless there has been a missed fracture, impairment of function, imperfect treatment or care, then there is little likelihood of a successful settlement for the patient. Only recently the danger of mismanagement of a small fracture was documented in the report of the Canadian Medical Protective Association (1978).

A 41-year-old tool-and-die maker, after twisting his ankle playing soccer, was treated in an Emergency Room, where the physician found no evidence of fracture on x-rays of the foot which he had ordered. He diagnosed the injury as a sprain of the ankle or foot and treated it accordingly with strapping. The following day a radiologist reviewed the foot films and reported them as showing no fracture although subsequently (and only in retrospect), a fracture through the lateral malleolus was visible in one view. Four days after the injury, the patient saw his family physician. This doctor was in touch with the hospital, confirmed that x-rays had been negative and referred the patient for physiotherapy. Weeks later, when the foot continued to be painful, an orthopedic surgeon saw the patient in consultation. He too called the hospital for a report, was told the x-rays showed no evidence of fracture and applied a short-leg walking cast for a month. He was not aware that x-rays were of the foot and not the ankle; he did not see the films nor did he order new x-rays. When the plaster was removed and when symptoms continued for some time, a second surgeon who saw the patient ordered x-rays, discovered the fracture which now showed callous formation and advised a period of physiotherapy without weight-bearing. The patient, now dissatisfied with the advice he was receiving, contacted an orthopedic surgeon who admitted him to hospital and ultimately, five months after the original injury, carried out a bone-grafting procedure from which the patient made a satisfactory recovery despite some superficial wound infection.

Three months after the plaster had been removed following the bone-grafting procedure there was some continuing swelling of the ankle and apparently because the patient was having difficulty in obtaining suitable

> *employment an orthopedic surgeon then in attendance provided the patient with a medical certificate indicating that sedentary employment would be desirable. On the advice of a provincial rehabilitation officer and on the basis of this certificate the patient was accepted for academic training in business administration so he might qualify for sedentary work. Some months later and apparently after there had been improvement, the same orthopedic surgeon wrote, "It will take him approximately one year from his surgical procedure to recover and after that he should be able to return to almost full activities." By this time the patient had been retrained.*
>
> *When a legal action was brought, liability had to be acknowledged because of the failure to detect the fracture which should have been recognized on the original x-ray films. Trial was necessary because of what seemed to be unreasonable financial demands of the plaintiff; the issues at trial were confined to those relevant to an assessment of damages.*
>
> *The court relied heavily on the opinion of the surgical expert who had not seen the patient but who gave his opinion that had the plaintiff been placed in a cast initially, he probably would have recovered without a permanent disability. On that basis, the court found that the plaintiff was entitled to an allowance for loss of income, past and future, because his earning capacity had been reduced and the plaintiff was awarded total damages of $86,162.18! Although the judgment was appealed, the appeal was unsuccessful, [Pp. 15–17]*

A costly error indeed.

The legitimate grievances, and the ones that cause us the most concern, are the result of preventable complications—acts of malpractice (errors of commission) or negligence (errors of omission). In such cases there is seldom any doubt in the patient's mind about the need for redress. Nor will there be any difficulty finding a lawyer to handle the case, for in many cases, the error is obvious—*res ipsa loquitor*—"the thing speaks for itself." The wrong eye or kidney has been removed, amputation of a limb followed the injection of drugs in an arm, mental retardation resulted from an anesthetic, or a foreign body was inadvertently left behind. Neither the patient's right to pursue legal action nor the lawyer's motives can be held in question. Nor can we complain if large awards are granted by judges and juries in such instances.

In the "gray" area of negligence, there are increasing numbers of legal actions. These involve errors in diagnosis, questionable postoperative management, inadequate follow-up of patients. Many of these have already been discussed. They are largely preventable errors, and again surgeons cannot blame their patients for seeking compensation for them. The reasons for the errors lie within us (the surgeons), and we should examine ways in which we can correct or prevent them.

THE LITIGATION-PRONE SURGEON

Just as there are litigious-minded patients, there are litigation-prone surgeons; and when two are brought together, the result may be foreordained. Just as there are common personality profiles among patients who sue, so too can we recognize personality patterns among surgeons who are sued. Such a surgeon may be contemptuous of his or her patients, referring to them as "cranks," "kooks," or "nuts." He or she may ignore or be insensitive to their complaints, especially pain. Such a surgeon may assume divine omniscience and omnipotence in front of patients. "This is one of the most common faults of surgeons with whom I have been involved in litigation," a lawyer once told me. "They take the attitude that they can do no wrong and challenge your right to question them." They are often evasive and communicate poorly with their patients. This air of infallibility can only engender hostility when something goes wrong, or even when it doesn't.

Such surgeons tend to guarantee success, a 100 percent cure; they promise that "you will look better, feel better;" They sound like a commercial for razor blades. This can be a dangerous practice, as they may later be sued for *breach of warranty,* particularly in the field of plastic surgery. Awards in the United States have been made where there was no negligence, but rather a breach of contract to achieve the condition promised by the operation.*

Of only less importance as a precipitating factor in litigation is a surgeon's lack of warmth, compassion, tact, sensitivity, whatever. As we have seen in the case of the retained foreign bodies, 42 percent of patients did not sue their surgeon even though they were aware of the retained foreign matter. This surely says something for communication and understanding between those patients and their surgeons. The C. M. P. A. has observed and warned its members repeatedly that the patients most likely to sue a doctor are those who feel that the doctor has slighted or neglected them or is lacking in interest or concern for their welfare.

How may surgeons recognize if they are litigation prone? A surgeon's recognition of dangerous personal traits is as important as recognizing the patient who may become a litigant. Any surgeon who is overconfident, overly self-assured, too hasty, or too rough can expect an increased incidence of complications and, possibly, a higher number of malpractice suits. A surgeon who is too quick to operate

---

*Gilbert Sharpe and Glenn Sawyer, *Doctors and the Law* (Toronto, Butterworth, 1979), p. 151.

without establishing a diagnosis, who fails to double-check X rays and tests, may have a tendency to extend his or her indications for surgery and, in fact, may perform unnecessary operations. A surgeon whose diagnostic accuracy is low and whose willingness to operate is high may have difficulty justifying these inconsistencies in a malpractice suit.

Such a surgeon tends to be casual about keeping records or operative reports, and his or her follow-up notes on patients are inadequate. An operative report dictated three months after an operation is meaningless, and the surgeon's memory is easily challenged and often found wanting by an astute lawyer in court.

Surgeons who are constantly operating on the fringes of their specialties and encroaching on those of others are asking for trouble. Today, with modern communication and travel, there is no excuse except situations of extreme urgency for a surgeon to perform an operation in a specialty in which he or she has had little training or experience. If those endeavors should result in tragedy, the surgeon must accept the blame. The surgeon who operates in several hospitals, practices itinerant surgery, or is constantly signing out to colleagues on weekends may someday be charged with surgical abandonment, for it is difficult to supervise the postoperative care of one's patients personally when they are scattered about in different communities and institutions. The conscience of the surgeon must form an integral part of the humane practice of surgery.

In summary, the vulnerable surgeon is superconfident, a supersalesperson who pushes patients to surgery. Such a surgeon is too quick to operate and operates too quickly. These faults result in unnecessary surgery, inadequate workups, faulty diagnosis, carelessness, removing the wrong part, leaving foreign bodies behind.

Some surgeons in this category think that once they have performed the operation, everything will go well afterward. They fail to follow up patients in the postoperative period and frequently leave their care to residents, or they sign out to other surgeons. This abandonment in the critical postoperative period can have tragic consequences, as we have seen.

It has been estimated that one in four surgeons in the United States will eventually be sued. This means, of course, that the majority (three of four) will not be. It is among the small group who will be sued that we must search for ways to improve.

THE LAWYER

More than a specific act of negligence or malpractice involving a surgeon toward a patient is required to institute a suit. Another important actor in this medicolegal drama, perhaps the most important person of all, is the lawyer. With the high-percentage contingency fees in the United States and the monumental awards given by judges and juries everywhere, malpractice litigation has become a highly lucrative field for the enterprising lawyer.

A survey by the National Association of Insurance Commissioners (and reported by Charlotte I. Rosenberg in *Medical Economics*) revealed that the average award to a successful claimant was up 28 percent between 1976 and 1978. The New York Insurance Department reports that awards and settlements against New York doctors rose from $20,796,000 in 1976 to over $40 million in 1978.*

A malpractice lawyer has been called "a frustrated surgeon who can't stand the sight of blood." As a simple solution to the problem of malpractice, others have suggested that we simply do away with lawyers. Do away with

---

*Charlotte L. Rosenberg, "Why a New Malpractice Crisis Is Coming," *Medical Economics*, October 29, 1979, pp. 109–114.

lawyers? Impossible, you say. Consider, however, that Japan, a country with a population of about 90 million more people than in Canada, for example, has only 10,000 lawyers. Why there are nearly that many lawyers in the province of Ontario alone. But lawyers and the adversary system, like death and taxes, are here to stay.

Do malpractice lawyers, like patients and surgeons who are prone to sue and be sued, have common traits? Of course it is dangerous to generalize, but many see themselves as knights in shining armor, protecting the innocent (patient) against the dragon (surgeon) of incompetence. They tend to see a black or white act of guilt or innocence in every malpractice situation, without any gray areas of doubt. Many fail to appreciate the subtleties of diagnosis, the importance of instant judgment in emergency, life-and-death situations. To them, every case is a "screw-up," and the majority of doctors, "bungling incompetents." Though this may be an overexaggeration when applied to all lawyers, this is what Stanley Rosenblatt, famous U.S. malpractice lawyer, has to say about doctors (in *People* magazine, September 1978): "I basically do not like them. It's due in part to their training. They become tin gods, with the attitude of how dare anyone question them. They will almost never admit they made a mistake." He states that he takes cases on a contingency basis. "If I win, I get between 25 and 40 percent of the verdict." His solution to the problem is simple: "The medical profession should police itself. Damn it, they know who the bad surgeons are, who does the unnecessary surgery, who shows up drunk or unprepared. But do they do anything about it? No. They're cover-up specialists."

This brings us to the contingency fee system, a widespread practice in the United States. Many consider it to be one of the prime reasons for the increase in malpractice suits in this country—the larger the award, the higher the lawyer's fee. Lawyers do well by malpractice awards.

Dr. Robert A. Fischl wrote in the *New England Journal of Medicine:* "Who has become the most important person in the practice of medicine aside from the doctor and his patient? Not the patient's relatives, not the nurse, not the technician; it is the lawyer. The inescapable fact is that the legal profession has encroached into the practice of medicine." He feels that this has not improved patients' welfare but hurt it. "We must get these lawyers off our backs, get them to take care of their own crisis, the crisis in their profession, the crisis of politics in the federal government." The lawyer–doctor relationship is not always a mutual admiration society.

THE JUDGE AND JURY

Not all judges are totally unbiased, as most of them are former lawyers. A judge of the Supreme Court of California stated, "The doctor is the party best able to protect himself through insurance, if the result of a procedure is not perfect or acceptable. The physician should be required to pay no matter whose fault it is—it is irrelevant to prove negligence or to search for negligence in the assessment of claims, but that payment should be made in any event for any untoward complication." Here is a judge who demands perfection of doctors and insists on awards for any "untoward" complication. How should we define "untoward?" Unexpected? Unpleasant? Unlucky? Unfortunate? Unfavorable? Inexpedient? To use the words "any untoward complication" for the myriad of unavoidable, inherent complications shows a basic failure to grasp the complexities of medicine and surgery. Perhaps someone should pay, and perhaps patients should be compensated for "untoward" complications, but that someone need not always be the physician.

It is understandable that the sympathies of juries (if not judges as well) are usually with the injured plaintiff.

This partly explains the magnitude of awards. It is a simple progression from surgical complications to negligent surgeon to commensurate compensation. A member of a jury can more readily identify with the patient (plaintiff) than with the surgeon (defendant). But higher and higher awards foster more and more malpractice suits, mounting insurance premiums, and higher and higher surgical fees—in the United States, at any rate. One New York jury awarded a plaintiff $800,000 for a mispositioned belly button; an out-of-court settlement reduced the figure to $200,000 on appeal. And malpractice insurance, though more readily available than a few years back through the formation of insurance companies by doctors themselves and by the activation of joint underwriting associations (JUAs) by individual states, is costly; indeed, some doctors (though not many) are not insured at all—called "going bare."

Let us examine how the system operates at the present time in the United States. How does a patient with a legitimate grievance seek redress? First he or she goes to a lawyer. The lawyer weighs the evidence pro and con and decides whether there is reasonable likelihood of success. (Malpractice lawyers, in Canada at least, only take from 10 to 40 percent of cases brought to them.) Before deciding, a lawyer may seek expert medical opinion from a friend or acquaintance and may write the doctor or surgeon a letter asking for an explanation of the complication. He or she probably will write the hospital medical records department for copies of the history, operative report, pathology report, and final note. These documents must be released to the lawyer, with the patient's signed release.

The surgeon who receives a letter from a lawyer (or from the medical records department to the effect that patient information has been requested), often panics and becomes defensive and paranoid. In the United States, doctors are advised to go immediately to their insurance carrier to have the matter handled properly. Recently formed malpractice insurance companies that are owned by doctors work hard to resolve such problems out of court, and thus to keep costs down. When the doctor-owned insurance company believes the patient has just cause to seek compensation, it offers a settlement that may well be satisfactory to the claimant. It often will be satisfactory to the insurance company, too, however, because it is lower than it would have been if it had had to include the amount the lawyer would have charged for pleading the case in court.

When such an offer is not forthcoming, however, lawyer and plaintiff have some time to decide whether to pursue the matter. The time allowed varies from state to state. In New Jersey, for example, the law allows a plaintiff two years from the date of discovery of the alleged injury to file a law suit. A plaintiff who was a minor when an alleged medical malpractice occurred has two years beyond the age of majority to file a suit. The time lag allowed is defined by the statute of limitations for each state and works for the benefit of the plaintiff. It can be a year of hell for the doctor, knowing of all the legal activity that is going on, wondering whether he or she will be sued.

And who pays for all this? Why the patient pays—through increased medical costs that have been raised to cover the price of medical malpractice insurance, of course. And who suffers? Not the lawyer, to be sure; the patient, perhaps; the doctor, certainly. Who profits? Why the lawyer, of course! And if he or she pursues the client's case and wins an award, the lawyer's reward will be handsome indeed.

Mr. Rosenblatt, the lawyer quoted earlier, who charged a 25 to 40 percent contingency fee, won an award for a client of $338,000. At the lower rate, this amounts to a fee of $84,000, and $135,000 at the higher figure. And this final amount was settled out of court! Even surgeons cannot help but be impressed by these figures. Let us now examine ways in which these disasters may be avoided.

10 How to reduce malpractice suits

Dr. Joseph F. Sadusk of George Washington University wrote a paper entitled "A Primer for Avoiding Malpractice Suits." In it he lists a number of commandments directed to the physician. They are equally applicable to surgeons.

1. *Give every patient scrupulous care.*

2. *Avoid unethical criticism of the work of other surgeons.*

3. *Keep complete records.*

4. *Make no statement that might be construed as an admission of fault on your part.*

5. *Exercise tact as well as professional ability in handling patients and insist on professional consultation if you have doubts about diagnosis or treatment, or if the patient or his family seem dissatisfied with your efforts.*

6. *Refrain from over-optimistic prognoses.*

7. *Notify patients of any intended absences from practice and recommend a qualified substitute to serve in your place.*

8. *Get, without fail, an "informed consent" (preferably in writing) for any surgical procedures and for autopsy.*

9. *Carefully select and supervise assistants and take care in delegating to them only those duties for which they are qualified.*

10. *Keep abreast of general medical and scientific progress.*

11. *Limit your practice to those fields that are well within your qualifications.*

12. *Make every effort to reach an understanding with your patient, about fees, preferably in advance of treatment.*

13. *Except in emergency situations, avoid examining a female patient unless an assistant nurse is present.*

14. *Exhaust all reasonable methods of securing a diagnosis before embarking on a therapeutic course.*

15. *Use conservative and the least dangerous methods of diagnosis and treatment whenever possible.*

These are commandments directed to the individual surgeon or doctor. Can anything be done as a group to reduce malpractice claims?

IMPROVING STANDARDS

The most obvious thing is to continue efforts to improve standards of selection, training, and accreditation. This is being done continuously. The efforts of the American College of Surgeons have been most diligent and commendable in this direction. The college strongly recommends that patients choose their surgeons from among those who are certified by a surgical board approved by the American Board of Medical Specialties as well as being Fellows of the American College of Surgeons. The college produced four public information brochures in 1979 under the collective title: *When You Need an Operation;* their titles are as follows:

1. *"Who Should Do Your Operation?"*—*how to assess a doctor's qualifications.*

2. *"Giving Your Informed Consent"*—*emphasizes how important it is to understand what the surgical procedure entails and to discuss any areas of concern with the surgeon.*

3. *"What Will Your Operation Cost?"*—*lists kinds of expenses to expect and advises discussion of costs with the surgeon.*

4. *"Should You Seek Consultation (Second Opinion)?"*—*discusses conditions under which getting additional advice may be a good idea.*

These are available to your doctor from the American College of Surgeons.

It is a difficult thing to wipe out incompetence completely. And it is impossible to legislate away errors and ineptitude. The governing bodies of surgery must continue in their attempts to reduce unnecessary surgery, to eliminate ghost surgery and itinerant surgery. Surgeons as a group must be made aware of the trend toward mandatory second opinion programs and should be prepared to accept them and to participate as peer experts when asked to give a second opinion. Unless we do so, we will become unwilling participants in the programs, and the resultant damage to our public image (already tarnished) will be considerable. Or we may find that legislators and insurance companies will take the matter out of our hands completely by making second opinions mandatory.

Another way to reduce the incidence of unnecessary surgery within a hospital is to have more effective tissue committees with regulations that have meaning rather than merely paying lip service to hospital accreditation requirements. This is the only way that medical advisory boards within community hospitals can control the performance of unnecessary surgery and the incidence of marginally unnecessary procedures. If we are to respond to charges that we are too tolerant of incompetents, then there is no alternative but to police ourselves.

Some groups do police themselves. In New Jersey, for example, the Bergen County Medical Society has a Committee on the Impaired Physician. Doctors are encouraged to turn over to the committee any information they may have about physicians whose performance is obviously impaired—whether it be through alcoholism, drug addiction, emotional instability, whatever. The committee then handles the matter with the physician in question discreetly. Doctors are motivated to keep impaired physicians from treating patients not only to protect the patients but also to protect the reputation and accreditation of the hospital(s) with which they themselves are affiliated. Impaired physicians do not make good impressions.

Regular death rounds or death committees must become part of the ongoing, in-hospital review system to determine the cause of deaths and find ways to minimize or prevent them. This area has for too long been deemphasized within hospitals. If such systems are not provided within by the surgical staff, then we can expect that others will provide them from without. Presently, unexplained deaths are investigated by the local coroner and/or medical examiner. The system varies from state to state. In Bergen County, New Jersey, for example, the medical examiner, working with the prosecutor's office, has the authority to investigate all deaths that occur within twenty-four hours of admission to a hospital; those that occur suddenly or unexpectedly; all deaths that are apparent homicides, suicides, or accidents; and deaths that occur in the work place or that are a threat to public health. But deaths from negligence, incompetence, poor judgment, unnecessary surgery, and the like usually escape official attention. I'm not suggesting more outside review but that we review more of them ourselves. Death rounds, like tissue committees, should form an intrinsic part of quality control for the consumer (patient).

We should look into ways to set up no-fault insurance for patients. This can be provided by doctors themselves (such as was done with P. S. I.), as is being done by groups of physicians in Florida. Or it might be issued by hospital organizations (e.g., Blue Cross) and underwritten by insurance companies. In this way, a patient who experiences unanticipated pain, suffering, or economic hardship from an unavoidable (inherent) complication of an operation could be redressed. There would be no need for litigation. This is not to say that the adversary system should be eliminated, not at all.

No-fault insurance would provide a minimum level of compensation for *all* victims (such as no-fault car insurance plans or workmen's compensation) and not solely for the victims of malpractice or negligence. At present there is no system for awarding sufferers of minor or moderate injuries short of a malpractice action, which may be too costly to undertake and may result in failure or no award at all.

For those complications considered to be preventable, where malpractice or negligence seems involved, or where large awards are being demanded, the courts would continue to serve as final arbiter. Undoubtedly, though, the legal lobby against no-fault insurance would be enormous.

MEDICOLEGAL PANELS OF ARBITRATION

Who would decide into which category a complication would fall? Who would determine what was inherent risk and what was avoidable injury? For this, it would be necessary to establish medicolegal panels of arbitration. A committee of two doctors, two lawyers, and two laypersons might screen claims to decide their merits and who should pay—the insurance company under no-fault insurance, or the surgeon's medical malpractice insurance by court decision. Such a committee might decide that there is no ground for any claim at all and thereby reduce the number of nuisance claims considerably.

This would give everyone a fair preliminary hearing—patients and doctors—and relieve the burden in the courts. The panelists could be chosen by the Bar Association, the College of Physicians and Surgeons, or the Medico-Legal Society. Such a panel would be a simple extension of the complaint and discipline committees of the medical and legal societies, though it would not in fact discipline but would arbitrate instead.

Such panels presently exist in the States of New York, Pennsylvania, Ohio, Illinois, California, and several others. The Province of Ontario, Canada, has studied these plans, and a committee recommended *against* their adoption. In Pima County, Arizona, the committee consists of nine doctors and nine lawyers. Many areas using such plans testify to their effectiveness and to the general satisfaction with them of the medical and legal associations.

It is unlikely, in the United States at least, that government (consisting mainly of lawyers) will ever legislate against contingency fees, but surely some ceiling should be put on these. Their continued existence can only serve to encourage unscrupulous lawyers to seek higher awards for their clients.

The outlook on another potential means of reducing nuisance claims in the future—the countersuit—is dim. According to Charlotte Rosenberg: "In state after state, the courts have quashed countersuits, reversing earlier victories and refusing to let other such suits be tried. With the decline of the countersuit movement—doctors' great hope only a few years ago against meritless malpractice suits—plaintiff's attorneys these days are being emboldened to file more and more malpractice suits [p.110]."* The purpose of such countersuits would not be to recover court costs that would have been charged to the plaintiff. Rather, the purpose would be to recover damages for loss of time, inconvenience, unnecessary harassment, and possible injury to one's professional reputation.

PATIENT SELF-HELP

Patients can help to reduce the number of unnecessary malpractice actions. The first way is by not having unreasonable expectations for surgery. Surgery is merely a therapeutic tool, not a miraculous be-all and end-all for humanity's ailments. By recognizing that there are inherent risks in any operation and that, indeed, the individual patient may be the greater risk, the person undergoing an operation is less likely to blame the surgeon for every untoward complication. By careful selection of your surgeon, hospital, and anesthesiologist, you may reduce your risk considerably and thereby avoid a tragedy.

It merits repeating that the qualities you should look for in your surgeon, apart from training and qualifications, are warmth, sincerity, dedication, and a willingness to communicate. When there is doubt about your diagnosis, the need for surgery, or the type of operation planned, insist on either a second opinion or more information. To be a party to informed consent, you must be informed, both verbally and in writing.

As a patient, you can demand no-fault insurance for unanticipated complications for which your surgeon cannot

---

*Charlotte L. Rosenberg, "Why a New Malpractice Crisis Is Coming," *Medical Economics,* October 29, 1979, pp. 109–114.

be held responsible. The public can urge the medical and legal bodies to set up panels of experts to screen claims and thus avoid unnessary legal fees and nuisance claims that have little chance for success.

The most important factor is that there be communication, meaningful dialogue between patient and surgeon. That is the surest way to achieve harmony and a climate for an optimum surgical result.

Index

Abortion, 2–3
A/C (aorto/coronary bypass), 36, 42–43, 64
Accidents, in hospital, 50–51
Accreditation, hospital, 40, 52–53
Acute care unit (ACU), 103–4, 106, 107
Admission, 76–78
Ambulation, early, 108
American Board Examinations, 36
American Board of Medical Specialties, 138
American College of Surgeons (ACS), 26, 28–29, 37, 38, 41, 139
    Fellows of, 36, 138–39
    Surgical Education and Self-Assessment Program of, 47
Anesthesia, 91–93
    agents of, 92
    errors with, 95–99
Anesthesiologists:
    meeting, 86–88
    in operating room, 91–93

Annals of Surgery, 26
Antibiotics, 51, 90
Appendectomy, 10, 56, 73
Arbitration, 141–43
Assisting surgeons, 80–83
Atropine, 90
Awards, in malpractice suits, 132, 133, 135

Bed capacity, 52, 75–76
Bergen County Medical Society, 140
Bladder, postoperative complications and, 70
Blood specimens, 77
Blue Cross/Blue Shield, 50, 73, 141
Board certification, 36–37
Bowel cancer, 30, 65
Bowel functions, postoperative, 109, 112
Bowel operations, 10, 106
Breach of warranty, 130
Breast augmentation, 11–12
Breast surgery, 12, 13, 64–65

Brewster, Kingman, 115
Bulletin of the American College of Surgeons, 55, 56, 115–16

Canadian Medical Protective Association (C.M.P.A.), 13–16, 18–22, 69, 84, 96–100, 126–28, 130
Cancer operations, 1, 10, 12, 30–31, 64–65
Cancer surgeons, 35
Cardiac surgeons, 35
CAT (computerized axial tomography), 18
Catheters, 105–6, 109–10
Cesarean section, 2
Chest X ray, 77, 87
Cholecystectomy, 73
Cleveland Clinic, 42, 43
Clinical judgment of surgeon, 62
Compassion of surgeon, 62
Complication rate review, 55–58
Consent, 11, 66–67, 78–85, 88, 119–25
Contingency fees, 133, 142
Coronary-artery bypass, 39
Coronary-artery disease, 1, 64
Cosmetic surgery, 2, 11–12, 35, 73–76
Coughing, postoperative, 107–8, 113
Craniotomy, 36

D & C (dilatation and curettage), 13, 27
Death rounds, 140–49
Deferral of operation, 78
Depression, postoperative, 112
Diagnosis, 17–33
  certainty about, 30–33
  establishment of, 17–25
  uncertainty about, 25–30

Diagnosis errors, 129
Diagnostic acumen of surgeon, 62
Digit, reimplantation of, 12
Dissection, 93–94
Doctors and the Law (Sharpe and Sawyer), 83
"Doctor's surgeons," 42
Drains, 105, 107, 110
Duodenal ulcer operations, 64

Ectopic pregnancy, 10
EKG, 77, 87
Elective surgery, 9–12, 26–30, 73–76
Emergency surgery, 1–2, 8–10
Endotracheal intubation, 91–92, 104–5
Equipment use, malpractice suits and, 39
Esophagus operations, 106
Execution, errors of, 99–100
Expectations, unreasonable, 118, 126–28, 143
Experience of surgeons, 38–39

Facilities, hospital, 49
Family physicians, as sources of information, 40–43, 46
Fees:
  lawyer, 133, 142
  surgeon, 35–36, 45, 73–74
Fee splitting, 45
Fellows of the American College of Surgeons, 36, 138–39
Fellows of the Royal College of Surgeons, 38
Fetal distress, 10
Fischl, Robert A., 134
Friedman, Meyer, 61
Friends, as sources of information, 45

Gallbladder operations, 10, 12, 27, 39–40, 56, 66, 78, 100, 110
Gallstone operations, 10, 30, 31, 64
Gas cramps, 109
Gas machine, 92
Gastric operations, 39, 100, 106
Gastric tube, 106, 107, 109
Gastrointestinal surgeons, 34
General anesthetic, 16
General-practitioner (GP) surgeon, 34, 36–37, 48
"Ghost" surgeons, 44–45
GI tract, postoperative complications and, 70
Group practice, 41
Guide to Hospital Accreditation, 57
Gynecologic surgery, 27
Gynecologists, 31–35

Handicapped surgeons, 43–44
Health Information Foundation, 48
Heart, postoperative complications and, 71
Heart operations, 1, 10, 36, 42–43, 64
Hernia operations, 10–11, 29–33, 56
Hip fractures, 9
Hospital costs, 3, 49–50
Hospitals:
  choosing, 48–58
    accreditation, 40, 52–53; cost and, 49–50; facilities, 49; medications, errors in, 50–51; mortality and complication review, 55–58; size, 48; staff compatibility, 53–55

  the operation, 89–102
    anesthesia, 91–93; anesthetic errors, 95–99; preliminaries, 89–91; process of, 93–95; surgical errors, 99–102
  postoperative period in, 103–14
    common reactions, 111–12; complications, 113–14; departure, 112–13
  preoperative period in, 75–88
    admission, 76–78; anesthesiologist, 86–88; preadmission, 75–76; written consent, 78–85, 88
Houston Clinic, 43
Hunter, John, 5
Hysterectomy, 2, 9, 10, 12, 27, 28, 56, 68–69, 73

Incision, 93
  closure of, 94–95
  postoperative complications and, 70
Infections:
  acquired in hospital, 51
  preoperative treatment of, 71–72
  risk of, 65–66, 68
Informed consent, 11, 66–67, 82–85
Ingrown toenail operations, 15–16
Inherent risk, 69–72, 126
In-service examinations, 38
Instrument counts, 101
Insurance, 29, 50, 73
  malpractice, 3, 116, 135–36
  no-fault, 3–4, 141, 143–44
Intensive care unit (ICU), 103–7
Interns, as sources of information, 46
Intravenous line, 106

Joint Commission on Accreditation of Hospitals (JCAH), 52
Joint underwriting associations (JUA), 135
Judges, 134
Judgment, errors in, 99
Juries, 134–35

Kidneys:
  operations on, 110
  postoperative complications and, 70

Lahey Clinic, 40, 49
Laparotomy, 56
Lawsuits (*see* Malpractice suits)
Lawyers, 132–36
Limbs:
  postoperative complications and, 70
  reimplantation of, 12
Litigation (*see* Malpractice suits)
Litigation-prone surgeons, 129–32
Litigious patients, 116–29
Liver operations, 106
Lungs:
  operations on, 10
  postoperative complications and, 70

Magnitude of operation, 12–16
  discussion with surgeon about, 64–65
Major surgery, 12–13
Malpractice, defined, 72
Malpractice insurance, 3, 116, 135–36
Malpractice suits, 2, 3, 5, 9, 115–44
  against anesthesiologists, 86
  awards, 132, 133, 135
  consent and, 119–25
  diagnosis and, 18–25, 32–33
  equipment use and, 39
  judges, 134
  juries, 134–35
  lawyers, 132–36
  litigation-prone surgeons, 129–32
  litigious patients, 116–29
  minor surgery and, 13–16
  negligence and, 19, 69, 72, 100–102, 129
  process of, 135–36
  reduction of, 137–44
    commandments for surgeons, 137–38;
    improving standards, 138–41; medicolegal panels of arbitration, 141–43;
    patient self-help, 143–44
  unreasonable expectations and, 118, 126–28, 143
Massachusetts General Hospital, 43, 49
Mastectomies, 12, 64–65
Matas, Rudolph, 61
Mayo Clinic, 40, 43, 49, 80
Medicaid, 50, 73
Medical Economics, 132
Medic Alert necklace or bracelet, 76–77
Medicare, 50, 73
Medications, errors in, 50–51
Medicolegal panels of arbitration, 141–43
Mental handicaps of surgeons, 43–44
Minor surgery, 13–16
Mortality rates, 39–40, 67–68
  review of, 55–58

Index

Motor vehicle accidents, 1, 118–19
Muscle relaxant, 92

Nasogastric tube, 106, 107, 109
National Association of Insurance Commissioners, 51, 132
Necessity of operation, 63–64
Negligence, 19, 69, 72, 100–102, 129
Neurosurgeons, 34, 35
Neurosurgery, 35
New England Journal of Medicine, 134
New York Insurance Department, 132
No-fault insurance, 3–4, 141, 143–44
Nolen, William A., 42–43
Nurses:
  notes of, 111
  as sources of information, 45–46

Ochsner Clinic, 49
Omission, errors of, 100–102
Operating room, 90–91
Operation, the, 89–102
  anesthesia, 91–93
  anesthetic errors, 95–99
  preliminaries, 89–91
  process of, 93–95
  surgical errors, 99–102
  (*see also* Surgery)
Ophthalmologists, 35
Orthopedic surgeons, 34
Orthopedic surgery, 9, 12, 27
Otolaryngologists, 35

Pancreas operations, 36, 40, 106
Patient self-help, 143–44

Patients' Rights Act of 1977, The (Ontario), 84
Pediatric surgeons, 35
Physical examination:
  in hospital, 77
  by surgeon, 63
Physical handicaps of surgeons, 43–44
Plastic surgery, 2, 11–12, 35, 73–76
Pneumonia, postoperative, 71, 113
Postoperative period, 103–14
  common reactions, 111–12
  complications, 113–14
  departure, 112–13
Preadmission, 75–76
Preoperative period in hospital, 75–88
  admission, 76–78
  anesthesiologist, 86–88
  preadmission, 75–76
  written consent, 78–85, 88
Preventable complications, 69–70, 72–73
Prostate operations, 27

Qualifications of surgeons, 36–37

Reconstructive operations, 12
Referring physicians, as sources of information, 40–43
Residents, 111
  as sources of information, 46
  surgery by, 80–83
Res ips loquitor principle, 69–70, 81, 129
Results of surgeons, 38, 39–40
Retina, operations on, 12
Risks of operations, 65–74
  inherent, 69–72, 126

Risks of operations, *continued*
  preventable complications, 69–70, 72–73
Rosenberg, Charlotte L., 132, 142–43
Rosenblatt, Stanley, 133
Rosenman, Ray H., 61

Sadusk, Joseph F., 137
St. Michael's Hospital, Toronto, 29, 53
Sawyer, Glenn, 67, 87
Scott, Charles F., 84
Second opinion, 25–30, 63
Self-assessment exams (SESAP), 47
Self-confidence of surgeons, 60–61, 62
Semimajor surgery, 12–13
Semiurgent surgery, 10
Sentinel effect, 28
Settlements, 132
Sharpe, Gilbert, 67, 87
Shouldice Clinic, Toronto, 52
Sleeplessness, postoperative, 112
Smith, W. D., 62
Soul of the Surgeon, The (Matas), 61
Sponges, lost, 100–101
Staff compatibility, 53–55
Standards, improving, 138–41
Status Report on Professional Liability, A, 116
Stee, Virgil, 56
Stomach operations, 39, 100, 106
Surgeons:
  assisting, 80–83
  characteristics of, 60–63
  choosing, 34–47
    criteria for, 35–40; practical approaches to, 40–45; sources of information to avoid, 45–46
  consent and, 78–85
  discussion topics with, 63–74
    fees, 73–74; magnitude, 64–65; necessity, 63–64; preventable complications, 69–70, 72–73; risks, 65–74; unpreventable or unavoidable complications, 69–72
  experience of, 38–39
  fees of, 35–36, 45, 73–74
  general-practitioner (GP), 34, 36–37, 48
  "ghost," 44–45
  handicapped, 43–44
  litigation-prone, 129–32
  in postoperative period, 111
  qualifications of, 36–37
  results of, 39–40
  staff compatibility, 53–55
  training of, 37–38
  varieties of, 34–35
Surgery, 8–33
  cosmetic, 2, 11–12, 73–76
  diagnosis, 17–33
    certainty about, 30–33; establishment of, 17–25; uncertainty about, 25–30
  elective, 9–12, 26–30, 73–76
  emergency, 1–2, 8–10
  magnitude of, 12–16, 64–65
  major and semimajor, 12–13
  minor, 13–16
  semiurgent, 10
  urgent, 10
  (*see also* Hospitals; Surgeons)
Surgical errors, 99–102
Sutures, 94–95
  removal of, 110

Team surgery, 80
Technical errors, 99–100

Technical expertise of surgeon, 62
Tests, hospital, 76–78
Thoracic surgeons, 35
Tissue committee, 55–58, 139–40
Tonsillectomy, 13
Tonsils, 56
Training of surgeons, 37–38
Tranquilizer, 90
Trussell Report, 37, 48
Tubal ligation, 12
Type A personality, 61–62

Unavoidable complications, 69–72
Unforeseeable complications, 126
Unnecessary surgery, 2, 41, 56
Urgent surgery, 10
Urinary fistula, 69

Urine specimen, 77
Urologic surgeons, 34, 35

Varicose veins, 10
Vasectomy, 12
Vein ligation, 56

Weight loss:
    postoperative, 112
    preoperative, 71
When You Need an Operation,
    139
Work, return to, 113
Wound infection, risk of, 65–66, 68

X rays, 18, 77, 87